Neonatal OSCE

Beyond the Books

Neonatal OSCE
Beyond the Books

Srinivas Murki
DM (Neonatology) MD (Pediatrics)
Chief Neonatologist
Paramitha Children Hospital, Kothapet
Hyderabad, Telangana, India

Rhishikesh Thakre
DM (Neonatology) MD (Pediatrics)
DNB DCH FCPS MBBS FIAP FNNF
Neonatal Consultant
Neo Clinic
Chhatrapati Sambhaji Nagar
Maharashtra, India

Foreword
Praveen Kumar

JAYPEE

JAYPEE BROTHERS MEDICAL PUBLISHERS
The Health Sciences Publisher
New Delhi | London

Jaypee Brothers Medical Publishers (P) Ltd

Headquarters
EMCA House, 23/23-B
Ansari Road, Daryaganj
New Delhi 110 002, India
Landline: +91-11-23272143,
+91-11-23272703
+91-11-23282021, +91-11-23245672
e-mail: jaypee@jaypeebrothers.com

Corporate Office
4838/24, Ansari Road, Daryaganj
New Delhi 110 002, India
Phone: +91-11-43574357
Fax: +91-11-43574314
e-mail: jaypee@jaypeebrothers.com

Overseas Office
JP Medical Ltd.
83, Victoria Street, London
SW1H 0HW (UK)
Phone: +44-20 3170 8910
e-mail: info@jpmedpub.com

EU GPSR Authorised Representative
Logos Europe, 9 rue Nicolas Poussin
17000, La Rochelle, France
Phone: +33 (0) 6 67 93 73 78
e-mail: contact@logoseurope.eu

Website: www.jaypeebrothers.com
Website: www.jaypeedigital.com

Neonatal OSCE Beyond the Books

First Edition: 2025

Reprint: 2026

ISBN 978-93-6616-651-3

Printed in India

Dedication

To the newborns, who teach us to be strong;
we cheer you on every single day.

To their parents, who overcome the trials of neonatal care
through never ending hope, patience and faith in us.

To our spouses and children who provide
unwavering support, making the journey possible
for those of us called to this work.

Preface

The journey to excellence in Neonatology demands a blend of knowledge, hands-on skills, assured clinical judgment, and effective communication—all of which are rigorously assessed through the Objective Structured Clinical Examination (OSCE). As a comprehensive, standardized, and universally recognized tool, the OSCE objectively evaluates clinical competencies and plays a central role in competency-based medical education (CBME). Beyond its function as an assessment method, it is also a powerful teaching modality, providing an effective framework for gauging the clinical proficiency of medical students and trainees.

This book, *Neonatal OSCE: Beyond the Books*, is designed as a thorough and targeted guide for those striving to excel in OSCEs while developing practical neonatal skills. It presents a wide range of cases and structured scenarios covering key areas in neonatal medicine—including history taking, physical examination, resuscitation, essential newborn care, emergency management, test interpretation, clinical procedures, research, and counseling.

Recognizing that the OSCE challenges both skill and composure, this book is designed to provide readers with not only the technical expertise but also the confidence to tackle each case with clarity and competence. We have organized the content to be practical and user-friendly, incorporating case-based examples and insights that reflect the variety and complexity of situations encountered in neonatology. With this approach, our goal is to help learners not only succeed in OSCEs but also deepen their understanding of neonatology and strengthen their proficiency in real-world clinical practice.

We hope this book will be an invaluable resource for residents, fellows, and practicing neonatologists alike, providing them with the knowledge, confidence, and skills necessary to excel in their examinations and, more importantly, in their clinical practice to deliver compassionate, effective care to neonates and their families.

Srinivas Murki
Rhishikesh Thakre

Foreword

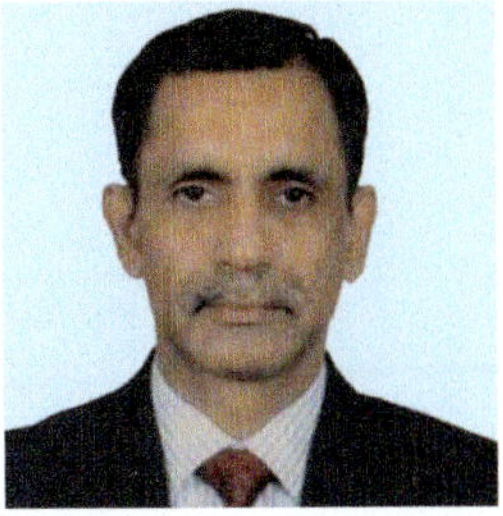

Practical training in medicine, especially in a specialty like Neonatology, is not at all an easy task. For the safety and comfort of vulnerable neonates, as well as for ethical reasons, the trainees need to practice with structured and simulated scenarios, rather on real patients. Objective Structured Clinical Examination (OSCE) is one of the most commonly used standard tools to train as well as assess the students in the application of clinical knowledge, judgement, and skills. There are very few resource materials related to OSCEs in neonatology.

Drs Rhishikesh Thakre and Srinivas Murki, two of the top neonatology teachers in the country, have come out with yet another excellent practical book *Neonatal OSCE: Beyond the Books* in their efforts to improve and standardize training in neonatology. They are most sought after and enthusiastic teachers of neonatology in the country, and have trained thousands of postgraduates, fellows and nurses over the years. They have decades of practical, hands-on experience of taking care of a variety of small and sick neonates, as well as establishing neonatal care units. They have the expertise and experience of developing exam questions including OSCEs and evaluating the trainees.

This masterly easy-to-read book should be of immense help to students of neonatology at all levels—postgraduates, fellows, DNB, DM as well as nursing students, as well as their teachers. The authors cover the most common clinical situations likely to be encountered by the neonatology trainees. The structure of the case scenarios covers elicitation of history, targeted physical examination, essential investigations, management as well as counseling.

I am sure this book will become an essential part of the study material for all students of neonatology.

Praveen Kumar DM (Neo) MD
Professor and Head
Division of Neonatology
PGIMER, Chandigarh, India

Acknowledgments

We wish to acknowledge Shri Jitendar P Vij (Group Chairman) and Mr Ankit Vij (Managing Director), Ms Chetna Malhotra (Senior Director - Professional Publishing, Marketing, and Business Development) of M/s Jaypee Brothers Medical Publishers (P) Ltd, New Delhi, India for their support and expertise in publication of this book. Their dedication to excellence and commitment to bringing this work to life have been instrumental in its creation.

Special thanks to Naman Singh, Development Editor for his commitment and support.

Contents

Section 6 Clinical Skill

Section 7 Counseling

Section 8 Miscellaneous

SECTION 1

History Taking

CHAPTER 1.1

History Taking

Setting: You are a resident on call. This patient is brought by parents for ________.

TASK

- Take history from the caregiver.
- Summarize and provide a provisional diagnosis.
- Lay down plan for action.
- You are not required to examine the patient.

DURATION

10 minutes

CHECKLIST

Step	*Tick here*
Approach: • Wash hands, ensure asepsis as required • Introduce self and role • Confirm patient identity • Explain you are here to take history details • Gain consent for history taking	
Chief/presenting complaint: Use open questioning to describe caregivers' chief complaint	
History of present illness	
• *Onset:* Day of life • *Mode:* Acute, subacute, and chronic • *Duration:* Hours, days, and weeks • *Progress:* Features of severity or complications • Associated complaints, if any • Ask for risk factors • *Time course:* Progression, response, and therapy • Explore caregiver ideas, concerns, and expectations (ICE) • Summarize for caregiver to confirm, correct, or modify any information	

Contd...

Contd...

Step	***Tick here***
Systemic enquiry: *Ask for relevant history:* Birth, perinatal, past illness, medication, family, diet, social, and so on	
Closing: • Summarize for caregiver and ask if any information is missed • Thank the caregiver for the time	
Summary: • Summarize with name, age of the patient, presenting complaint, and relevant medical history • Make a provisional diagnosis or offer a differential diagnosis	
Communication skills	
• Caregiver friendly language • Open/closed questioning • Active listening, understanding, and empathy • Fluency • Rapport with caregiver • Nonverbal communication • Summarizing	

TIPS

- Use open questioning to explore problem and its details.
- Rephrase question to gain more clarity.
- Provide enough time to caregiver for answering details.
- Do not interrupt caregivers' narrative.
- Report in caregivers' language.
- Use focused question to ensure specific information.
- Show nonverbal cues—eye to eye contact, sit at level of caregiver, nodding, facial expressions, hand gestures, and uninterrupted attention.
- Ensure privacy.

CHAPTER 1.2

Excessive Crying

Setting: You are in the outpatient department (OPD). A day 40, baby is brought to you by parents for excessive crying. Ask history that will aid you in diagnosis and management.

OBJECTIVE

At the end of history taking in an infant with excessive crying one should be able to reach following conclusions:

- Is it a well-baby or sick baby?
- What is the onset, duration, and progress?
- Are there any clues to the underlying cause?
- Is it physiological or pathological?

BACKGROUND

Excessive crying in early infancy is common. Most of the times, it is transient and self-limiting. It poses significant stress to the parents and doctors. It is important to identify normal from abnormal crying.

PRESENTING COMPLAINT

Use open questioning to identify the chief complaints.

"What concern do you have for the baby?"
"What do you think is wrong with the baby?"

Open questioning enables the parent to describe their concerns. Listen attentively and avoid interruptions.

HISTORY OF PRESENTING COMPLAINT

It is important to identify the onset, duration, and progress (ODP).

- *Since when is the baby crying?*
- *Could you describe the crying episode?*
- *Is the crying episode for the first time or does it happen repeatedly?*

Ask questions that will help to define *how the baby is between the episode* of excessive crying.

- *How is the feeding pattern—normal, decreased, or absent?*
- *How is the activity pattern—normal, decreased, or absent?*
  Ask focused questions that will help *define the etiology* of excessive crying.

Perinatal

- *Did the baby cry at birth or needed help?*
- *Did the baby have any illness requiring hospitalization?*
- *What is the baby's birth weight? Current weight?*

Feeding

- *Does the baby respond to feeding?*
- *How is the baby fed—mother's milk or formula or top milk?*
- *What is the color of urine, frequency of urine and stool?*
- *Is there vomiting or poor stool passage?*

Infection

- *Does the baby have noisy breathing?*
- *Does the baby have fever, rash, foul umbilicus, feeding difficulty, or fast breathing?*
- *Is there any abnormal movement or body posture?*
- *Is there any ear discharge?*
- *Does the baby move all limbs or not?*

SYSTEMIC REVIEW

- Is there bluishness noticed on crying?
- Is there vomiting or poor stool passage?
- Is the vomitus green or stool red?
- Is the baby appropriately dressed?

Family

- *Does any family member have fever, cough, and cold?*
- *Does anybody smoke in the house?*

GENERAL ENQUIRY

- *What is your occupation, workplace?*
- *What is the home address, and details of family members?*
- *Who cares for the baby? How is the mother's response?*
- *Did you do anything to treat the baby so far?*
- *Are maternal concerns different from paternal?*

EXPLORE CAREGIVER IDEAS, CONCERNS, EXPECTATIONS

- *What are your thoughts on the problem?*
- *What's your major worry regarding the problem?*
- *What do you think should be plan of action?*

SUMMARIZING

Provide a concise overview of the information the parent has shared regarding their current issue. This step ensures you have an accurate grasp of the patient's medical history and allows them to rectify any inaccuracies. After summarizing, inquire if there are any additional details you might have missed, and maintain periodic summaries as you proceed through the remaining medical history.

CLOSING THE SESSION

Ask the parent if they have any questions or concerns that have not been addressed. Thank the parents for their time.

CONCLUSION

Male child of Babi, day 40 old, born at term gestation, 2.6 kg birth weight with uneventful delivery is brought by parents for excessive crying. The baby is well prior and in between the episodes, exclusively breastfed, with no perinatal or postnatal risk factors, with normal colored urine and stool with past similar episodes.

Most probably, it appears to be physiologic due to infantile colic.

I would like to examine the baby to confirm my clinical impression and plan investigations, if required.

Clinical Reasoning

1. *Is the baby well or sick?*
   How the baby is prior to episode or between the episodes provides clue to the wellbeing. A well-baby is playful in between the episodes with good feeding and sleep. A sick baby has poor feeding and sleep and remains irritable in between.
2. *How is the onset, duration and progress?*
   Abrupt onset, first episode crying suggests an acute problem which may be physiological or pathological. Recurrent episodes in a well-baby may suggest physiological cause like infantile colic but in a baby with poor weight gain it points to pathology.
3. *What is the underlying cause?*
   Perinatal:
   - History of asphyxia, home delivery, prematurity-related complications or any illness requiring neonatal intensive care unit (NICU) stay may predispose to acute crying episodes, e.g., sequalae to asphyxia, sepsis, severe jaundice, intraventricular hemorrhage, hemorrhagic disease of the newborn (HDN), and chronic lung disease.

- Birth weight and current weight provides trend of wellness of the baby. Weight loss >7% of birth weight or >3% daily indicates inadequate intake and is pathological.
- Feeding should soothe the baby if it is hungry. Baby not responding to feed usually indicates nonhunger causes.

Postnatal:

- Adequacy of lactation is indicated by frequent and clear urination; baby being contented after feed and sleeps postfeed. High-colored urine indicates inadequate lactation and high-colored urine staining the diapers indicates direct jaundice. Top fed baby must have enquiries to dilution used and mode of feeding. Bottle feeding may predispose to flatulence, gastrointestinal (GI) infection, or ear infection.
- Infections such as sepsis, pneumonia, meningitis, acute otitis media, umbilical sepsis, or osteomyelitis present with excessive crying. Such infants are not well in between the episodes.
- Repeated vomiting, poor stool passage suggest GI problem. GI infection or obstruction may cause green vomitus and or red stool.
- Crying leading to cyanosis suggest cyanotic heart disease and or unconsolable crying could occur due to supraventricular tachycardia
- Hypo or hyperthermia may cause discomfort.

Family history:

- A family member with upper respiratory tract infection (URTI) may also cause similar illness with blocked nose in the baby.
- Cigarette smoking is irritating and avoidable in the household.
- Separated parents, single parent, nuclear family, and economic hardship put stress on the mother and may interfere with parenting role.
- Caretaker in absence of parents may not be responsive to the baby needs.
- Mother's indifference to baby crying may suggest drug abuse, illness, or depression.
- Varying or contradictory history or concerns by parents may suggest child abuse.

Acute Crying Checklist

Step	*Tick here*
Approach: • Wash hands, ensure asepsis as required • Introduce self and role • Confirm patient identity • Explain you are here to take history details • Gain consent for history taking	
Chief complaint: Use open questioning to describe caregivers' chief complaint	
History of present illness	
• Ask question to identify if the baby is well or sick • Ask for onset, duration, and progress • Ask for feeding details	

Contd...

Contd...

Step	***Tick here***
• Ask for risk factor—perinatal and postnatal • Ask caregiver ideas, concerns, and expectations (ICE) • Summarize for caregiver to confirm, correct, or modify any information	
Systemic enquiry: *Ask for relevant history:* Family, diet, social, immunization, and vitamin K injection at birth	
Closing: • Summarize for caregiver and ask if any information is missed • Thank the caregiver for the time	
Summary: • Summarize with name, age of the patient, presenting complaint, relevant medical history • Make a provisional diagnosis or offer a differential diagnosis	

CHAPTER 1.3

Admission of Preterm Infant at Birth to Neonatal Intensive Care Unit

Setting: A 32-week-old girl child of Ratna is being admitted from the delivery room. Take history that would aid your management.

OBJECTIVE

At the end of history taking, if a preterm infant is being admitted to the NICU, one should be able to reach the following conclusions:

- Is the baby symptomatic or asymptomatic?
- What risk factors predisposed to prematurity?
- Were prenatal steroids, magnesium sulfate and other preventive strategies practiced?

BACKGROUND

Prematurity is one of the common indications for admission to NICU. Babies born preterm may be asymptomatic or symptomatic and may have identifiable maternal risk factors. History often guides to cause of prematurity and helps lay down priorities in management.

Presenting Complaint

Use open questioning to identify the chief complaints.

"What concern do you have for the baby?"
"What do you think is wrong with the baby?"

Open questioning enables the parent to describe their concerns. Listen attentively and avoid interruptions.

HISTORY OF PRESENTING COMPLAINT

It is important to identify the onset, duration, associated symptoms, and progress (ODP) of any complaint the baby has.

- *When did you notice the baby to have difficulty (Note the age in hours)?*
- *Is the difficulty increasing or same or decreasing?*

- *Does the newborn have associated problems such as cyanosis, fast breathing, chest retractions, and audible sounds?*
- *Is the baby active or dull?*

Ask focused questions that will help *define the etiology* of prematurity.

Prenatal

- *What is the maternal age and gestational age?*
- *Was mother ANC registered? How many visits? Any medications? Any problem identified during pregnancy? Any problem in previous pregnancy? Interpregnancy interval?*
- *Was antenatal steroid given to mother—dose or course, complete, or incomplete?*
- *Was magnesium sulfate given to mother—complete or incomplete course?*
- *Did the mother have any diabetes, pregnancy-induced hypertension (PIH), antepartum hemorrhage, polyhydramnios, oligohydramnios?*
- *Was there any leakage or urinary tract infection (UTI) and was mother given any antibiotics?*
- *Was any prenatal scan done and were there any concerns?*

Intrapartum

- *How was the mode of delivery—vaginal or C section?*
- *Did the mother have fever, leaking, lower abdominal pain, foul discharge, or UTI?*
- *Was the liquor clear or meconium stained?*
- *Was there any sentinel event (cord prolapse, bleeding, fetal heart changes, decreased fetal movements, and excess or low liquor volume)?*

Postnatal

- *Did the baby cry at birth or needed help?*
- *What is the baby's birth weight?*

Ask for *family history* to seek clues to cause of respiratory distress (RD).

- *Is there family history of prematurity?*
- *Is this a consanguineous marriage?*

General Enquiry

- *What is your occupation, home place?*
- *What is the home address, and details of family members?*
- *What is social, economic, and educational background?*

Explore Caregiver Ideas, Concerns, and Expectations

- *What are your thoughts on the problem?*

- *What's your major worry regarding the problem?*
- *What do you think should be plan of action?*

Summarizing

Provide a concise overview of the information the parent has shared regarding their current issue. This step ensures you have an accurate grasp of the patient's medical history and allows them to rectify any inaccuracies. After summarizing, inquire if there are any additional details you might have missed, and maintain periodic summaries as you proceed through the remaining medical history.

CLOSING THE SESSION

Ask the patient if they have any questions or concerns that have not been addressed. Thank the parents for their time.

Clinical Reasoning

- *Is the preterm baby symptomatic or asymptomatic?*
  Babies born preterm may have one or more of the following symptoms at birth—RD, grunt, fast breathing, apnea, decreased cry, or activity. It suggests a systemic problem. Many preterm infants may be asymptomatic on admission but go on to develop problems with passage of time.
- *How is the onset, duration, and progress?*
  Respiratory distress is the most common problem in preterm at birth. In RD syndrome (RDS), congenital pneumonia, and meconium aspiration, the onset is at birth and the severity worsens with time. In transient tachypnea of newborn (TTN), the onset is at birth but the severity may reduce with time. Aspiration, pneumothorax, pneumonia, lung malformations, and heart diseases may present with RD later and may progress over time.
- *What is the underlying cause?*

Prenatal:

- Poor prenatal care, short interpregnancy interval, underage, elderly, poor weight gain during pregnancy, obesity, multiple pregnancy, infertility treatment, complicated medical disorders, and cervical or uterine problems predispose to preterm labor
- Use of prenatal steroids in babies <34 weeks gestation accelerates lung maturity reducing the incidence and severity of RDS, need for invasive respiratory support, oxygen duration, hospital stay, and improving survival. The benefits of steroids extend to other common morbidities in preterm, viz., intraventricular hemorrhage (IVH), patent ductus arteriosus (PDA), circulatory instability, and necrotizing enterocolitis (NEC).
- Magnesium sulfate provides neuroprotection for infants born below 32 weeks of gestation.
- Maternal illness such as diabetes may increase risk of RDS, persistent pulmonary hypertension of the newborn (PPHN), and malformation in the newborn. PIH contributes to intrauterine growth restriction (IUGR), perinatal asphyxia, and secondary RDS/PPHN and TTN.

- Premature rupture of membranes may result in chorioamnionitis, preterm labor, and early delivery.
- Polyhydramnios may occur with uncontrolled maternal diabetes and congenital diaphragmatic hernia (CDH).
- Fever, rash, and lymphadenopathy may suggest congenital infections (TORCH).

Intrapartum:
- Abruptio placenta and placenta previa may precipitate preterm labor and lead to aspiration of blood and secondary RDS.
- Chorioamnionitis may trigger onset of labor and result in congenital pneumonia.
- Difficult delivery is suggested by precipitate labor or prolonged labor delivery predisposing to birth trauma, asphyxia leading to RD.

Postnatal:
- Weak cry or absent cry, need for resuscitation at birth indicates perinatal asphyxia. Asphyxia may serve as additional burden to premature immature organs.
- Infant of diabetic mother (IDM) and preterm are at risk of RDS

Family History
- Previous sibling with prematurity or family history of prematurity is the most common cause of preterm labor.
- Consanguineous marriage predisposes to genetic or inborn errors of metabolism. Surfactant protein B deficiency may be inherited as autosomal recessive disorder.
- Low educational status, poor economic background, and socially backward predispose to multiple etiologies of preterm labor.

CONCLUSION

A 32-week-old girl child of Ratna, 30 minutes of birth is admitted for preterm care. The baby is born to primi, registered with five antenatal care (ANC) visits brought in emergency for bleeding per vaginum due to placenta previa with mild PIH, single dose of dexamethasone being given with no dose of magnesium sulfate given and delivered by C-Section. The baby cried at birth and currently is asymptomatic with very low birth weight and would need continuous monitoring and ongoing care.

Preterm Admission Checklist

Step	*Tick here*
Approach: • Wash hands, ensure asepsis as required • Introduce self and role • Confirm patient identity • Explain you are here to take history details • Gain consent for history taking	
Chief complaint: Use open questioning to describe caregivers' chief complaint	

Contd...

Contd...

Step	*Tick here*
History of present illness:	
• Ask question to identify problem, if any • Ask for onset, duration, and progress • Ask for risk factors—prenatal, natal, and postnatal • Ask for steroid and magnesium sulfate coverage • Ask for leakage, maternal urinary infection, and antibiotic usage • Ask caregiver ideas, concerns, and expectations (ICE) • Summarize for caregiver to confirm, correct, or modify any information	
Systemic enquiry: Ask for relevant history: family, diet, social, and immunization.	
Closing: • Summarize for caregiver and ask if any information is missed • Thank the caregiver for the time	
Summary: • Summarize with name, age of the patient, presenting complaint, and relevant medical history • Make a provisional diagnosis or offer a differential diagnosis	

CHAPTER 1.4

Not Gaining Weight

Setting: This day 16 boy born at 36 weeks is brought by parents for concerns of inadequate weight gain. Ask for relevant history to guide your management.

OBJECTIVE

At the end of history taking in an infant with concerns of weight, one should be able to reach following conclusions:

- Is weight loss subjective or objective?
- Is feeding adequate or inadequate?
- Is the problem with the mother or with the baby?
- What is the underlying cause?

BACKGROUND

Birth of a preterm baby is a nutritional emergency. Late preterm and very preterm babies are at risk of extrauterine growth restriction due to inadequate feeds due to immaturity or illness. All infants should have growth assessment at every opportunity postdischarge. Lactational inadequacy or problems with the baby may come in the way of adequate weight gain. Babies lose weight during first 7–10 days if term and up to 14 days if preterm. One should be able to identify if the weight loss is pathological and what is the underlying cause.

PRESENTING COMPLAINT

Use open questioning to identify the chief complaints.

- *"What concern do you have for the baby?"*
- *"What do you think is wrong with the baby?"*

Open questioning enables the parent to describe their concerns. Listen attentively and avoid interruptions.

Identify if the weight loss is subjective or objective.

- *Why does the mother feel weight gain is not adequate?*
- *Are there any loose skin folds?*
- *Does the baby appear small compared to its weight at birth?*

HISTORY OF PRESENTING COMPLAINT

It is important to identify that the onset, duration, and progress (ODP) of:

- *Since when did you first notice problem with weight of the baby?*
- *Has the baby weight taken since birth?*
- *What is the weight trend?*

Ask focused *feeding*-related questions.

Feeding History

- *Type of feeds*: Breast milk or formula or animal milk
- Number of times/24 hours, night feeds
- *If breastfed:*
  - Demand/scheduled feeding/switching breasts between feeds
  - Maternal breast or nipple problems such as sore nipples
  - *Method of feeding*: Direct/paladai
- *If formula/animal milk:*
  - Dilution
  - *Method of feeding:* Paladai/bottle
  - Type of formula

Pattern of feeding: Does baby feed well/poorly (sick child)/frantic sucking (hyperthyroidism)/suck rest suck?

Adequacy of Feeds

- *Urine output:*
  - Number of wet diapers per day (indicator of hydration status and polyuria)
  - Color of urine (concentrated/smoky for urine infection/urate crystals)
- *Stool pattern:*
  - Number of stools per day
  - Consistency of stools—normal semisolid/pellet like/loose stools (adequacy of feeds/infection/malabsorption)

Sleep: Duration of sleep after each feed

ASK QUESTIONS TO DEFINE THE UNDERLYING CAUSE

Prenatal

- *What is the gestational age?*
- *Was there any fetal distress (bradycardia, tachycardia, meconium liquor, Doppler abnormality, nonstress test, or continuous fetal monitoring abnormality)?*
- *Was the mother suffering from any other illness or on drugs during or before pregnancy?*

- *Was there any fever, rash, or lymphadenopathy during pregnancy?*
- *Was there any medical problem identified during pregnancy?*
- *Was there any history of polyhydramnios?*

Intrapartum

- *How was the mode of delivery—normal or C section?*
- *Was there any difficulty in delivery or prolonged labor?*
- *Did the mother have fever, leaking, lower abdominal pain, foul discharge, or urinary tract infection (UTI)?*

Postnatal

- *Did the baby cry at birth or needed help?*
- *Was the baby admitted after birth?*
- *Were any tests done on baby's blood—metabolic screen?*

Ask focused questions that will help define the *severity*.
- *How is the cry of the baby—normal, poor, or shrill?*
- *How is the activity pattern—normal, decreased, or absent?*

Ask for *family history* to seek clues.
- *Is there consanguinity of marriage?*
- *To which community do you belong (to find ethnicity)?*

General Enquiry

- *What is your occupation, workplace?*
- *What is the home address, and details of family members?*
- *How is the baby doing overall?*
- *Is the baby vaccinated?*

Explore Caregiver Ideas, Concerns, and Expectations

- *What are your thoughts on the problem?*
- *What's your major worry regarding the problem?*
- *What do you think should be plan of action?*

Summarizing

Provide a concise overview of the information the parent has shared regarding their current issue. This step ensures you have an accurate grasp of the patient's medical history and allows them to rectify any inaccuracies. After summarizing, inquire if there are any additional details you might have missed, and maintain periodic summaries as you proceed through the remaining medical history.

CLOSING THE SESSION

Ask the patient if they have any questions or concerns that have not been addressed. Thank the parents for their time.

Clinical Reasoning

- *Is weight loss subjective or objective?*
Many parents have concerns of weight due to crying baby, comparing with other babies or comments by relatives. Crying is thought to be due to feeding issue by majority. Crying may be due to hunger and beyond, e.g., boredom, soiling of diapers, passage of urine or stool, prior to sleep, and needing to be held, if the environment is too warm or cold or infantile colic. It may also suggest pain or hypoxia. Subjective feelings may be erroneous. Objective features to suggest weight loss are loose skin folds, ill-fitting clothes, loosening of bangle, and weight trend.
- *How is the onset, duration, and progress?*
Physiological weight loss takes place up to 7–10 days in term and up to 14 days in preterm infants. Any weight loss thereafter is pathological. Acute weight loss suggests poor intake while ongoing weight loss suggests underlying systemic pathology. Nutritional adequacy restores weight in majority. Non-nutritional causes such as systemic illness, metabolic, genetic, or an endocrine disorder are not restored on nutritional support only.
- *Is feeding adequate or inadequate?*
Adequacy of breastfeeding is judged by frequency and color of urine and stool, maternal breast fullness, and baby being contended after feed. Inadequate feeding leads to irritable baby, high colored urine, and mother feels less milk let down.
- *Is the problem with the baby or with the mother?*
Inadequate lactation suggests problem with the mother. It may be due to local breast problem or maternal illness or medications. Adequate lactation but poor weight gain suggests problem with the baby. It may be due to immaturity, oral pathology, recovery from illness, ongoing systemic diseases, or neglect.
- *What is the underlying cause?*

  Prenatal:
  - Very preterm/extremely low birth weight (ELBW), intrauterine growth restriction (IUGR) infants are likely to have inadequate weight gain due to multiple etiology.
  - Maternal illness, e.g., congenital infections (TORCH), diabetes, hypertension predispose to IUGR, prematurity, and IUGR thereby increasing risk for weight loss

  Intrapartum:
  - Fetal distress, difficult delivery, chorioamnionitis predisposes to asphyxia, sepsis, and prematurity thereby predisposing to poor weight gain.
  - C-section mothers have difficulty in feeding, need support and the babies are likely to be top fed.

  Postnatal:
  - Weak cry or absent cry, need for resuscitation at birth indicates perinatal asphyxia. Severe perinatal asphyxia leads to weight loss.
  - Weight loss >7% of birth weight or >3% daily indicates inadequate intake.

- Well at birth, adequate feeding, vomiting, and sudden onset seizures with encephalopathy may occur due to inborn errors of metabolism (IEM).

Family history: Consanguineous marriage predisposes to genetic or IEM that could result in poor weight gain.

CONCLUSION

Girl child of Pratiksha presents at 16 days of birth for parental concerns of poor weight gain. Baby was born at 35 weeks of gestation with maternal pregnancy-induced hypertension (PIH), birth weight of 2.4 kg and current weight of 2.5 kg. Baby cries a lot which leads to mother having concerns. The baby is exclusively breastfed and the history is suggestive of lactational adequacy. There are no features to suggest illness in the baby.

I would like to examine the baby to confirm my clinical impression and plan investigations, if required.

Not Gaining Weight Checklist

Step	*Tick here*
Approach: • Wash hands, ensure asepsis as required • Introduce self and role • Confirm patient identity • Explain you are here to take history details • Gain consent for history taking	
Chief complaint: Use open questioning to describe caregivers' chief complaint	
History of present illness	
• Ask question to differentiate subjective from objective weight loss • Ask for onset, duration, and progress • Ask for feeding details and feeding adequacy • Ask for risk factors—prenatal, natal, and postnatal • Ask caregiver ideas, concerns, and expectations (ICE) • Summarize for caregiver to confirm, correct, or modify any information	
Systemic enquiry: Ask for relevant history—family, diet, social, immunization, etc.	
Closing: • Summarize for caregiver and ask if any information is missed • Thank the caregiver for the time	
Summary: • Summarize with name, age of the patient, presenting complaint, and relevant medical history • Make a provisional diagnosis or offer a differential diagnosis	

CHAPTER 1.5

Jaundice

Setting: You are in the OPD. This day 3 baby is brought by parents for yellowish discoloration of the body. Ask relevant history to help you in management.

OBJECTIVE

At the end of history taking in an infant with jaundice, one should be able to reach following conclusions:

- Is the jaundice direct or indirect?
- What is the onset, duration, and progress of jaundice?
- Are there any complications due to jaundice?
- What is the probable underlying cause?

BACKGROUND

Jaundice is yellowish discoloration of skin, sclera, and mucosa. Jaundice in newborn becomes visible once the total serum bilirubin (TSB) is >5 mg/dL. Jaundice may be due to increase in concentration of direct bilirubin (conjugated hyperbilirubinemia) or indirect bilirubin (unconjugated hyperbilirubinemia) in the blood. It is important to identify jaundice, type of jaundice, its severity, and its etiology.

PRESENTING COMPLAINT

Use open questioning to identify the chief complaints.

- *"What concern do you have for the baby?"*
- *"What do you think is wrong with the baby?"*

Open questioning enables the parent to describe their concerns. Listen attentively and avoid interruptions.

Identify the *type of jaundice* by asking:

- *"How is the color of urine and stool"*

Urine staining the diapers or pale, or clay stool suggests conjugated jaundice. The discussion here shall be for unconjugated (indirect) jaundice.

HISTORY OF PRESENTING COMPLAINT

It is important to identify the onset, duration, and progress (ODP) of jaundice.

- *When did you first notice the baby to be yellow (Note the age in hours)?*
- *How many days since the baby is yellow?*
- *Is the jaundice same or increasing or decreasing?*
- *How is the feeding, sleep, and activity of the baby?*

Ask focused questions that will help *define the etiology* of jaundice.

Prenatal

- *What is the gestational age?*
- *What is the maternal gravida status?*
- *What is mothers blood group?*
- *Was the mother suffering from any illness or on drugs during or before pregnancy?*
- *Was there any problem identified during pregnancy?*
- *Was the mother's blood tested for human immunodeficiency virus (HIV), hepatitis B surface antigen (HbsAg), and Venereal Disease Research Laboratory (VDRL)?*

Intrapartum

- *How was the mode of delivery—normal or C section?*
- *Was there any difficulty in delivery or prolonged labor?*
- *Did the mother have instrumental delivery?*
- *Did the mother have fever, leaking, lower abdominal pain, or foul discharge?*
- *Was the liquor clear or meconium stained?*

Postnatal

- *Did the baby cry at birth or needed help?*
- *What is the baby's birth weight? What is the current weight?*
- *How is the baby fed—mother's milk or formula or top milk?*
- *What is the color of urine, frequency of urine, and stool?*
- *Does the baby have fever, rash, ear discharge, foul umbilicus, feeding difficulty, fast breathing, or abnormal movement?*
- *Were any tests done on baby's blood—metabolic screen?*
- *Do you know the baby blood group?*

Ask focused questions that will help define the *severity* of jaundice.

- *How is the feeding pattern—normal, decreased, or absent?*
- *How is the activity pattern—normal, decreased, or absent?*
- *How is the cry of the baby—normal, poor, or shrill?*
- *Is there any abnormal movement or body posture?*

Ask for *family history* to seek clues to cause of jaundice.

- *Is there consanguinity of marriage?*
- *To which community do you belong (to find ethnicity)?*
- *Are there any family members with jaundice?*
- *Do any members in mothers'/fathers' family side have blood disorders, blood transfusion, splenectomy, bile stones, or gallbladder removal?*
- *Did the previous sibling have jaundice requiring any therapy?*

General Enquiry

- *What is your occupation, workplace?*
- *What is the home address, and details of family members?*
- *How is the baby doing overall?*
- *Did you do anything to treat the jaundice so far?*
- *Is the baby vaccinated?*

Explore Caregiver Ideas, Concerns, and Expectations

- *What are your thoughts on the problem?*
- *What's your major worry regarding the problem?*
- *What do you think should be plan of action?*

Summarizing

Provide a concise overview of the information the parent has shared regarding their current issue. This step ensures you have an accurate grasp of the patient's medical history and allows them to rectify any inaccuracies. After summarizing, inquire if there are any additional details you might have missed, and maintain periodic summaries as you proceed through the remaining medical history.

CLOSING THE SESSION

Ask the patient, if they have any questions or concerns that have not been addressed. Thank the parents for their time.

CONCLUSION

Male child of Asha, 75 hours of age, born at term gestation, 2.6 kg birth weight with uneventful delivery is brought by parents for concerns of jaundice. The baby is well, exclusively breastfed, with no antenatal-intranatal or postnatal risk factors, with normal colored urine and stool with no setting for blood group incompatibility with jaundice up to abdomen as per parents with normal feeding pattern, cry, and activity.

Most probably it appears to be physiologic hyperbilirubinemia.

I would like to examine the baby to confirm my clinical impression and plan investigations, if required.

Clinical Reasoning

- *Is the jaundice direct (conjugated) or indirect (un-conjugated)?*
  Conjugated jaundice suggests hepatic, biliary, or hepatobiliary affection. It is always pathological, does not cross blood brain barrier, and merits urgent evaluation and treatment. Unconjugated bilirubin suggests increased breakdown of bilirubin. It may be physiological or pathological. It is potentially neurotoxic.
- *How is the onset, duration, and progress?*
  Early onset (<24 hours of age), prolonged (>14 days), and rapidly increasing jaundice suggests pathological jaundice.
- *Are there any complications?*
  Indirect bilirubin crosses the blood brain barrier and is neurotoxic causing bilirubin encephalopathy which manifests as alteration in sensorium, tone, cry, and activity. Conjugated jaundice may lead to liver cell failure and manifests as ascites, bleeding tendency, or encephalopathy.
- *What is the underlying cause?*

  Prenatal:
  - Preterm and late preterm are at risk for developing significant jaundice.
  - Primi is a risk factor due to increased risk of lactational inadequacy.
  - Mother with blood group O or Rh –ve status with baby A, B, AB blood group, or Rh +ve status respectively leads to blood group incompatibility.
  - Maternal illness such as diabetes, hypertension predispose to intrauterine growth restriction (IUGR), prematurity, and polycythemia thereby increasing risk for jaundice. Use of maternal oxytocin predisposes to neonatal jaundice due to altered red blood cell (RBC) osmolality of the fetus.
  - Congenital infections (TORCH) predispose to direct jaundice.

  Intrapartum:
  - Fetal distress by any mode of delivery predisposes to jaundice.
  - Difficult delivery is suggested by precipitate labor, prolonged labor, or instrumental delivery predisposing to birth trauma, asphyxia leading to jaundice in newborn
  - Maternal infection or fetal distress predisposes to significant jaundice in newborn.

  Postnatal:
  - Weak cry or absent cry at birth indicates perinatal asphyxia.
  - Weight loss >7% of birth weight or >3% daily indicates inadequate intake and is pathological.
  - Inadequate lactation predisposes to jaundice due to increase in enterohepatic circulation. Formula milk or use of top milk predisposes to infection, diarrhea, and dilution issues.
  - Adequacy of lactation is indicated by frequent and clear urination; baby being contented after feed and sleeps postfeed. High-colored urine indicates inadequate lactation and high-colored urine staining the diapers indicates direct jaundice.
  - Sickness predisposes to significant jaundice.
  - Metabolic disorders such as congenital hypothyroidism, galactosemia, cystic fibrosis, hemoglobinopathy, and glucose-6-phosphate dehydrogenase (G6PD) deficiency cause jaundice and can be detected by routine metabolic screening in a asymptomatic newborn.

- Mother with O blood group having a baby who is A, B, or AB blood group leads to ABO blood group incompatibility. Mother with Rh –ve blood group with a baby who is Rh +ve leads to Rh blood group incompatibly.

Family history:
- Consanguineous marriage predisposes to genetic or metabolic disorders such as hemoglobinopathy, G6PD deficiency, cystic fibrosis, and galactosemia predisposing to jaundice.
- Certain communities are at increased risk of hemoglobinopathy such as Parsis and Kutchis thereby higher prevalence of jaundice.
- F/h/o jaundice suggests hemolytic anemia, metabolic disorder, or inherited disorders of bilirubin metabolism.

Jaundice Checklist

Step	*Tick here*
Approach: • Wash hands, ensure asepsis as required • Introduce self and role • Confirm patient identity • Explain you are here to take history details • Gain consent for history taking	
Chief complaint: Use open questioning to describe caregivers' chief complaint	
History of present illness:	
• Ask question to identify type of jaundice • Ask for onset, duration and progress • Ask for feeding details • Ask for risk factors—prenatal, natal and postnatal • Ask for severity and complications • Ask caregiver ideas, concerns, expectations (ICE) • Summarize for caregiver to confirm, correct, or modify any information	
Systemic enquiry: Ask for relevant history—family, diet, social, immunization, etc.	
Closing: • Summarize for caregiver and ask if any information is missed • Thank the caregiver for the time	
Summary:	
• Summarize with name, age of the patient, presenting complaint, and relevant medical history • Make a provisional diagnosis or offer a differential diagnosis	

CHAPTER 1.6

Hypoglycemia

Setting: This baby at 6 hours after birth is brought to neonatal intensive care unit (NICU) for decreased feeding and activity. His dextrostix is 25 mg% on admission. Take relevant history for management of the case.

OBJECTIVE

At the end of history taking, in an infant with hypoglycemia one should be able to reach following conclusions:

- Is the baby symptomatic or asymptomatic?
- What is the onset, duration, and progress of hypoglycemia?
- Are there any complications?
- What is the probable underlying cause of hypoglycemia?

BACKGROUND

Hypoglycemia is the most common metabolic emergency. Hypoglycemia is a biochemical diagnosis and not a clinical diagnosis. All sick infants and "at risk" infants should have a glucose level done on admission. It is important to identify type of hypoglycemia, severity, and its etiology.

PRESENTING COMPLAINT

Use open questioning to identify the chief complaints.

- *"What concern do you have for the baby?"*
- *"What do you think is wrong with the baby?"*

Open questioning enables the parent to describe their concerns. Listen attentively and avoid interruptions.

Identify the *type of hypoglycemia* by asking:

- *"Is the baby having any symptoms or not?"*

Hypoglycemia may occur in a baby who is asymptomatic or with some symptoms. It is important to identify as the management approach differs.

HISTORY OF PRESENTING COMPLAINT

It is important to identify the onset, duration and progress (ODP) of hypoglycemia.

- *When did you first notice the baby to be not well (note the age in hours)*
- *How is the feeding, sleep, and activity of the baby?*

Ask focused questions that will help *define the etiology* of hypoglycemia

Prenatal

- *What is the gestational age?*
- *How was the weight gain in utero?*
- *What is the maternal gravida status?*
- *Was the mother suffering from any illness or on drugs during or before pregnancy?*
- *Was there any problem identified during pregnancy?*

Intrapartum

- *How was the mode of delivery—normal or C section?*
- *Was there any difficulty in delivery or prolonged labor?*
- *Did the mother have fever, leaking, lower abdominal pain, and foul discharge?*
- *Was the liquor clear or meconium stained?*

Postnatal

- *Did the baby cry at birth or needed help?*
- *What is the baby's birth weight? What is the current weight?*
- *How is the baby fed—mother's milk or formula or top milk?*
- *What is the color of urine, frequency of urine, and stool?*
- *Does the baby have fever, rash, ear discharge, foul umbilicus, or any feeding difficulty?*
- *Were any tests done on baby's blood—metabolic screen?*

Ask focused questions that will help define the *severity* of hypoglycemia.

- *How is the feeding pattern—normal, decreased, or absent?*
- *How is the activity pattern—normal, decreased, or absent?*
- *How is the cry of the baby—normal, poor, or shrill?*
- *Is there any abnormal movement or body posture?*

Ask for *family history* to seek clues to cause of hypoglycemia.

- *Is there consanguinity of marriage?*
- *Is there any unexplained neonatal deaths?*

General Enquiry

- *What is your occupation, workplace?*

- *What is the home address, family members?*
- *How is the baby doing overall?*
- *Did you do anything to treat the baby so far?*

Explore Caregiver Ideas, Concerns, and Expectations

- *What are your thoughts on the problem?*
- *What's your major worry regarding the problem?*
- *What do you think should be plan of action?*

Summarizing

Provide a concise overview of the information the parent has shared regarding their current issue. This step ensures you have an accurate grasp of the patient's medical history and allows them to rectify any inaccuracies. After summarizing, inquire if there are any additional details you might have missed, and maintain periodic summaries as you proceed through the remaining medical history.

CLOSING THE SESSION

Ask the patient if they have any questions or concerns that have not been addressed. Thank the parents for their time.

CONCLUSION

Male child of Asha, 6 hours of age, born at term gestation, 2.1 kg birth weight with uneventful delivery is brought by parents for concerns of decreased activity and poor feeding. The baby is drowsy with no antenatal-intranatal or postnatal risk factors with hypoglycemia documented on admission.

Most probably it appears to be symptomatic hypoglycemia in a small for gestational age (SGA) infant born to primi with unsupervised feeding and care.

I would like to examine the baby to confirm my clinical impression and plan investigations

Clinical Reasoning

- *Is there hypoglycemia?*
  The threshold for treating hypoglycemia in the first 4 hours is venous blood glucose values of <25 mg%, between 4 and 24 hours < 35 mg% and beyond 24 hours is <45 mg%.
- *Is the baby having symptomatic or asymptomatic hypoglycemia?*
  Asymptomatic hypoglycemia can be managed with supervised oral feeding but symptomatic hypoglycemia (e.g., lethargy, irritability, jitteriness, feeding difficulty, seizures, or apnea) needs intravenous glucose therapy.

- *How is the onset, duration and progress?*
Early-onset hypoglycemia (<72 hours) may be nutritional, metabolic, or perinatal stress induced while late-onset hypoglycemia (>72 hours) is likely to be sepsis or inherited metabolic disorders. Persistent (>7 days) or severe hypoglycemia (>12 mg/kg/min of glucose infusion rate) is secondary to inborn errors of metabolism, endocrine, storage disorder, or genetic cause. All these factors help in determining the etiology, management, and further investigations.
- *Are there any complications?*
Well baby but with risk factors for hypoglycemia e.g., SGA, large for gestational age (LGA), preterm, asphyxia, and infant of diabetic mother may be asymptomatic and hypoglycemia is detected only on screening. Presence of symptomatology suggests symptomatic hypoglycemia and warrants urgent intervention and has guarded prognosis. Abnormal odor of urine or body suggests metabolic disorder.
- *What is the underlying cause?*

Prenatal:
- Preterm and late preterm babies are at risk for developing hypoglycemia.
- SGA and LGA infants are predisposed to develop hypoglycemia.
- Primi is a risk factor due to increased risk of lactational inadequacy.
- Maternal illness such as diabetes, hypertension predispose to intrauterine growth restriction (IUGR), prematurity, and polycythemia thereby increasing risk for hypoglycemia. Use of maternal drugs (e.g., β-blockers, β2 agonists for tocolysis, salicylates, etc.) predisposes to neonatal hypoglycemia.

Intrapartum:
- Fetal distress, difficult delivery, precipitate labor, prolonged labor. or instrumental delivery predisposing to birth trauma, asphyxia causing hypoglycemia.
- Maternal infusion of dextrose during labor may cause rebound hypoglycemia in the newborn.
- Maternal infections causing sepsis manifests with hypoglycemia.

Postnatal:
- Weak cry or absent cry at birth indicates perinatal asphyxia.
- Weight loss >7% of birth weight or >3% daily indicates inadequate intake and is pathological suggesting lactational insufficiency.
- Adequacy of lactation is indicated by frequent and clear urination; baby being contented after feed and sleeps post feed. High-colored urine indicates inadequate lactation.
- Metabolic disorders such as galactosemia, hereditary fructose intolerance, and glycogen storage disorders cause hypoglycemia.

Family history: Consanguineous marriage or unexplained neonatal deaths suggest genetic or metabolic cause.

Hypoglycemia Checklist

Step	***Tick here***
Approach: • Wash hands, ensure asepsis as required • Introduce self and role • Confirm patient identity • Explain you are here to take history details • Gain consent for history taking	
Chief complaint: Use open questioning to describe caregivers' chief complaint	
History of present illness	
• Ask question to identify hypoglycemia and if the baby is symptomatic or asymptomatic • Ask for onset, duration, and progress • Ask for feeding details • Ask for risk factors—prenatal, natal, and postnatal • Ask for severity and complications • Ask for any odor to urine or body • Ask caregiver ideas, concerns, and expectations (ICE) • Summarize for caregiver to confirm, correct, or modify any information	
Systemic enquiry: Ask for relevant history: Family, diet, social, etc.	
Closing: • Summarize for caregiver and ask if any information is missed • Thank the caregiver for the time	
Summary: • Summarize with name, age of the patient, presenting complaint, and relevant medical history • Make a provisional diagnosis or offer a differential diagnosis	

CHAPTER 1.7

Respiratory Distress

Setting: You are in the ER. A term infant is brought at 2 hours of birth with increasing breathing difficulty. Ask relevant history to help you in your management.

OBJECTIVE

At the end of history taking in an infant with respiratory distress, one should be able to reach following conclusions:

- Is this respiratory distress?
- What is the severity of respiratory distress?
- What is the underlying cause?

BACKGROUND

Respiratory distress (RD) is tachypnea, recessions, and grunt with or without cyanosis. Severity of work of breathing as assessed by Silverman Anderson scoring or Downe's score, saturations, sensorium, and tone of the infants are used to assess severity of respiratory distress in newborn. Transient tachypnea of newborn, meconium aspiration pneumonia, pulmonary hypertension, and congenital pneumonia are the common causes of RD in term infants and RD syndrome (RDS) is the most common cause of respiratory distress in preterm infants. Congenital malformations of heart and lung could also present with RD in the newborn.

PRESENTING COMPLAINT

Use open questioning to identify the chief complaints.

- *"What concern do you have for the baby?"*
- *"What do you think is wrong with the baby?"*

Open questioning enables the parent to describe their concerns. Listen attentively and avoid interruptions.

When was this breathing difficulty noted and how is the progress?

HISTORY OF PRESENTING COMPLAINT

It is important to identify the onset, duration, associated symptoms, and progress (ODP) of respiratory distress.

- *When was it first noticed the baby to have difficulty in breathing (note the age in hours)?*
- *Is this breathing difficulty noticed from birth?*
- *Is the RD increasing or same or decreasing?*
- *Does the newborn have associated cyanosis, recessions, nasal flaring, and grunting?*
- *Is the baby active or dull? Did the baby become dull over time?*

Ask focused questions that will help to *define the etiology* of respiratory distress.

Prenatal

- *What is the gestational age?*
- *Was there any fetal distress [bradycardia, tachycardia, MSL, Doppler abnormality, nonstress test (NST) or contraction stress test (CST) abnormality]?*
- *Did the mother have any diabetes, pregnancy-induced hypertension (PIH), polyhydramnios, and oligohydramnios?*
- *Was targeted imaging for fetal anomalies (TIFFA) scan done?*
- *Was there any problem identified during pregnancy?*

Intrapartum

- *How was the mode of delivery—normal or C section?*
- *Was there any difficulty in delivery or prolonged labor?*
- *Did the mother have instrumental delivery?*
- *Did the mother have fever, leaking, lower abdominal pain, foul discharge, and urinary tract infection (UTI)?*
- *Was the liquor clear or meconium stained, or blood stained?*
- *Was there any sentinel event (cord prolapse, bleeding, fetal heart changes, decreased fetal movements, excess, or low liquor volume)?*

Postnatal

- *Did the baby cry at birth or needed help?*
- *What is the baby's birth weight? What is the current weight?*
- *How is the baby fed—mother's milk or formula or top milk?*
- *What is the color of urine, frequency of urine, and stool?*

Ask focused questions that will help define the *severity* of respiratory distress?

- *How is the sensorium normal, decreased, or irritable?*
- *How is the color, work of breathing?*
- *How is the cry of the baby—normal, poor, or shrill?*
- *How is the activity pattern—normal, decreased, or absent?*
- *How is the tone of the baby—normal, increased, and reduced?*

Ask for *family history* to seek clues to cause of respiratory distress.

- *Is there consanguinity of marriage?*

General Enquiry

- *What is your occupation, workplace?*
- *What is the home address, and details of family members?*
- *How is the baby doing overall?*
- *Is the baby vaccinated?*

Explore Caregiver Ideas, Concerns, and Expectations

- *What are your thoughts on the problem?*
- *What's your major worry regarding the problem?*
- *What do you think should be plan of action?*

Summarizing

Provide a concise overview of the information the parent has shared regarding their current issue. This step ensures you have an accurate grasp of the patient's medical history and allows them to rectify any inaccuracies. After summarizing, inquire if there are any additional details you might have missed, and maintain periodic summaries as you proceed through the remaining medical history.

CLOSING THE SESSION

Ask the patient if they have any questions or concerns that have not been addressed. Thank the parents for their time.

Clinical Reasoning

- *Does the newborn have respiratory distress or tachypnea?*
  Respiratory distress is presence of two of the three—(1) tachypnea, (2) recessions, and (3) grunt. Cyanosis is not component of definition. Infants with RD are more likely to have problems related to airway and lungs.
- *How is the onset, duration, and progress?*
  In RDS, congenital pneumonia, meconium aspiration syndrome (MAS) the onset is at birth and the severity worsens with time. In transient tachypnea of the newborn (TTN) the onset is at birth but the severity may reduce with time. Aspiration, pneumothorax, pneumonia, lung malformations, and heart diseases may present with RD later and may progress over time.
- *What is the severity of RD?*
  Infants with RD and dull, inactive, reduced tone, cyanosis, and increased work of breathing are more likely to have severe respiratory distress. Work of breathing is assessed by looking at recessions, nasal flaring, chest, and abdominal movements and grunt.

- *What is the underlying cause?*

  Prenatal:
  - The more immature the newborn, more likely the cause of RD is RDS. History of antenatal steroid coverage is also important as absent steroid coverage increases risk of RDS in preterm infants.
  - Maternal illness such as diabetes may increase risk of RDS, persistent pulmonary hypertension of the newborn (PPHN), and malformation in the newborn. PIH contributes to intrauterine growth restriction (IUGR), perinatal asphyxia and secondary RDS/PPHN and TTN.
  - TIFFA scan may identify congenital diaphragmatic hernia (CDH), malformations of lung, and heart
  - Polyhydramnios may occur with uncontrolled maternal diabetes, CDH, and lung malformations.
  - Fever, rash, and lymphadenopathy may suggest congenital infections (TORCH).

  Intrapartum:
  - Fetal distress by any mode of delivery predisposes to asphyxia and asphyxia lung injury, secondary RDS, and PPHN.
  - Abruptio placenta and placenta previa may lead to aspiration of blood and secondary RDS.
  - Chorioamnionitis may result in congenital pneumonia.
  - Difficult delivery is suggested by precipitate labor, prolonged labor or instrumental delivery predisposing to birth trauma, and asphyxia leading RD.

  Postnatal:
  - Weak cry or absent cry, need for resuscitation at birth indicates perinatal asphyxia.
  - Infants of diabetic mother (IDM) and preterm are at risk of RDS.
  - Fever, temperature instability, and late-onset RD may suggest pneumonia.
  - Tachypnea, high oxygen requirement may suggest CHD.

  Family history:
  - Consanguineous marriage predisposes to genetic or inborn errors of metabolism that could result in RD and RDS.
  - Surfactant protein B deficiency may be inherited as autosomal recessive disorder.

CONCLUSION

This newborn is presenting at birth and has a progress increase in RD. There is history of meconium staining of amniotic fluid and the baby was born by C section for fetal distress. The likely causes of RD in this baby are MAS and PPHN.

I would like to examine the baby to confirm my clinical impression and plan investigations, if required.

RESPIRATORY DISTRESS CHECKLIST

Step	*Tick here*
Approach: • Wash hands, ensure asepsis as required • Introduce self and role • Confirm patient identity	

Contd...

Contd...

Step	*Tick here*
• Explain you are here to take history details • Gain consent for history taking	
Chief complaint: Use open questioning to describe caregivers' chief complaint	
History of present illness	
• Ask question to differentiate RD from tachypnea • Ask for onset, duration, and progress • Ask for feeding details • Ask for prenatal TIFFA scan details • Ask for risk factors—prenatal, natal, and postnatal • Ask for steroid coverage in preterm deliveries • Ask for sensorium, vitals, and cyanosis • Ask caregiver ideas, concerns, and expectations (ICE) • Summarize for caregiver to confirm, correct, or modify any information	
Systemic enquiry: Ask for relevant history: Family, diet, social, immunization, etc.	
Closing: • Summarize for caregiver and ask if any information is missed • Thank the caregiver for the time	
Summary: • Summarize with name, age of the patient, presenting complaint, and relevant medical history • Make a provisional diagnosis or offer a differential diagnosis	

CHAPTER 1.8

Seizures

Setting: You are in the emergency room. This day 2, baby is brought by parents for abnormal body movements. Ask relevant history to guide your management.

OBJECTIVE

At the end of history taking in an infant with seizures, one should be able to reach following conclusions:

- *Is this a seizure or a seizure mimic?*
- *What is the type of seizure?*
- *What is the underlying cause?*

BACKGROUND

Seizures are the most common reason for emergency room visit of a newborn. Jitteriness, sleep myoclonus, hyperekplexia, and GER are the most common seizure mimics. Seizures are broadly categorized to automatisms, clonic, tonic, myoclonic, and autonomic seizures. Asphyxia, birth trauma/injury, metabolic disturbances, infections, infarcts/bleeds, inner ear malformation (IEM), and malformations are the most common causes of neonatal seizures. Early identification, classification, and etiology are useful to prevent further brain injury, manage and prognosticate. Always address temperature/airway/breathing/circulation (TABC) and control the seizures immediately before going for a detailed history and examination.

PRESENTING COMPLAINT

Use open questioning to identify the chief complaints.

- *"What concern do you have for the baby?"*
- *"What do you think is wrong with the baby?"*

Open questioning enables the parent to describe their concerns. Listen attentively and avoid interruptions.

Differentiate seizure by seizure-mimics by asking:

- *Is this movement spontaneous?*
- *How long it would last?*

- *Is this stimulus sensitive?*
- *Does it abort with restrain?*
- *Is it related to feeding?*
- *Does this appear only during sleep?*
- *Does the baby become blue, irritable, lose consciousness, and lose tone during or after the movement?*
- *Ask to enact the movement to define the semiology of seizure.*

HISTORY OF PRESENTING COMPLAINT

It is important to identify the onset, duration, and progress (ODP) of seizure/abnormal movement.

- *When did you first notice the baby to have this abnormal movements (note the age in hours)?*
- *Did you notice these movements from birth?*
- *How often and how long are these abnormal movements?*
- *Are the movements affecting upper limbs, lower limbs, eyes, mouth, and face? Are these movements symmetrical or focal?*
- *How is the feeding, sleep, and activity of the baby?*
- *During the abnormal movements how is the baby's activity, eye movements, mouthing movements, limb movements, color, and breathing?*
- *What happens to the baby immediately after the abnormal movement?* Ask focused questions that will help *define the etiology* of seizures.

Prenatal

- *What is the gestational age?*
- *Was there any fetal distress [bradycardia, tachycardia, meconium-stained liquor (MSL), doppler abnormality, nonstress test (NST), or contraction stress test (CST) abnormality]?*
- *Did the mother have any diabetes and pregnancy-induced hypertension (PIH)?*
- *Was the mother suffering from any other illness or on drugs (AEDs—antitubercular drugs) during or before pregnancy?*
- *Was there any fever, rash, or lymphadenopathy during pregnancy?*
- *Was there any problem identified during pregnancy?*
- *Was there any abnormal fetal movements?*

Intrapartum

- *How was the mode of delivery—normal or C section?*
- *Was there any difficulty in delivery or prolonged labor?*
- *Did the mother have instrumental delivery?*
- *Did the mother have fever, leaking, lower abdominal pain, foul discharge, and urinary tract infection (UTI)?*
- *Was the liquor clear or meconium stained?*

- *Was there any sentinel event (cord prolapse, bleeding, fetal heart changes, decreased fetal movements, and excess or low liquor volume)*

Postnatal

- *Did the baby cry at birth or needed help?*
- *What is the baby's birth weight? What is the baby's current weight?*
- *Did the baby receive vitamin K at birth?*
- *How is the baby fed—mothers' milk or formula or top milk?*
- *What is the color of urine, frequency of urine, and stool?*
- *Does the baby have fever, rash, ear discharge, foul umbilicus, feeding difficulty, and fast breathing?*
- *Were any tests done on baby's blood—metabolic screen?*

Ask focused questions that will help define the *severity* of seizures.

- *How is the sensorium after the abnormal movement—normal, decreased, or irritable?*
- *How is the cry of the baby—normal, poor, or shrill?*
- *How is the activity pattern—normal, decreased, or absent?*
- *How is the tone of the baby—normal, increased, and reduced?*
- *How is the color, breathing during and after the abnormal movement?*

Ask for *family history* to seek clues to cause of abnormal movement.

- *Is there consanguinity of marriage?*
- *To which community do you belong (to find ethnicity)?*
- *Are there any family members with seizures?*
- *Do any members in mothers/fathers family side have early infantile deaths, seizure disorder, developmental delays, and disabilities?*
- *Did the previous sibling have seizure requiring any therapy?*

General Enquiry

- *What is your occupation, workplace?*
- *What is the home address, and details of family members?*
- *How is the baby doing overall?*
- *Is the baby vaccinated?*

Explore Caregiver Ideas, Concerns, and Expectations

- *What are your thoughts on the problem?*
- *What's your major worry regarding the problem?*
- *What do you think should be plan of action?*

Summarizing

Provide a concise overview of the information the parent has shared regarding their current issue. This step ensures you have an accurate grasp of the patient's medical history and allows them to rectify any inaccuracies. After summarizing, inquire if there are any additional details you might have missed, and maintain periodic summaries as you proceed through the remaining medical history.

CLOSING THE SESSION

Ask the patient if they have any questions or concerns that have not been addressed. Thank the parents for their time.

Clinical Reasoning

- *Are the abnormal movements seizures or seizure mimics?*
  Seizures are spontaneous onset, not stimulus sensitive, cannot be restrained, associated with abnormal gaze, shrill cry, tachycardia, and desaturations. Post seizure the baby is usually dull, inactive and may be hypotonic. Jitteriness is stimulus sensitive, can be restrained and not associated with abnormal vitals. Sleep myoclonus is sudden jerky movements mostly occur during sleep and not during awake state.
- *How is the onset, duration and progress?*
  Seizures that present in the first 24–48 hours of birth are mostly due to asphyxia or birth injuries. Delayed onset may be due to infections, malformations, and metabolic errors. Seizures due to asphyxia, metabolic abnormalities are mostly transient and do not result in epilepsy.
- *What is the seizure semiology?*
  Enacting of seizures by parents or caregivers or a video recording is very useful to define the semiology of seizures. Seizures are broadly classified to automatisms, clonic, tonic, myoclonic, and autonomic seizures.
- *What is the underlying cause?*

  Prenatal:
  - Very preterm/very low birth weight (VLBW) infants are likely to have seizures due to multiple etiology.
  - Maternal illness such as diabetes, hypertension predispose to intrauterine growth restriction (IUGR), prematurity, and polycythemia thereby increasing risk for seizures.
  - Fever, rash, and lymphadenopathy may suggest congenital infections (TORCH).

  Intrapartum:
  - Fetal distress by any mode of delivery predisposes to asphyxia and seizures.
  - Chorioamnionitis may result in early onset sepsis, meningitis, and seizures.
  - Difficult delivery is suggested by precipitate labor, prolonged labor, or instrumental delivery predisposing to birth trauma, asphyxia leading to seizures in newborn.
  - Maternal infection or fetal distress predisposes to seizures in newborn.

  Postnatal:
  - Weak cry or absent cry, need for resuscitation at birth indicates perinatal asphyxia.
  - Infants of diabetic mothers (IDM), late preterm, and IUGR are prone for hypoglycemia, polycythemia, and hypocalcemia.

- Weight loss >7% of birth weight or >3% daily indicates inadequate intake and may be associated with polycythemia, hypoglycemia and venous thrombosis.
- Inadequate lactation especially in late preterm, IUGR, and IDM predispose to hypoglycemia and seizures
- Well at birth, adequate feeding, vomiting, and sudden onset seizures with encephalopathy may occur due to IEM.

Family history:

- Consanguineous marriage predisposes to genetic or inborn errors of metabolism that could result in neonatal seizures.
- Family of seizures could be present with familial myoclonic seizures, IEMs, and channelopathies (Na and K channel disorders).

CONCLUSION

Girl child of Manisha presents at 48 hours of birth. Baby was born at term with birth weight of 2.5 kg. Mother had history of PIH, baby was low birth weight and IUGR. Feeding was inadequate and baby lost 300 g from birth. From the video presentation, it seems to be clonic seizure. From the details of history, seizures appear secondary to be hypoglycemia.

I would like to examine the baby to confirm my clinical impression and plan investigations, if required.

SEIZURE CHECKLIST

Step	*Tick here*
Approach: • Wash hands, ensure asepsis as required • Introduce self and role • Confirm patient identity • Explain you are here to take history details • Gain consent for history taking	
Chief complaint: Use open questioning to describe caregivers' chief complaint	
History of present illness	
• Ask question to differentiate seizures from jitteriness and sleep myoclonus • Ask for onset, duration, and progress • Ask for feeding details • Ask for risk factors—prenatal, natal, and postnatal • Ask for sensorium, vitals, abnormal eye, and mouth movements • Ask for sensorium, tone, and movements after cessation of seizures • Ask caregiver ideas, concerns, and expectations (ICE) • Summarize for caregiver to confirm, correct, or modify any information	
Systemic enquiry: Ask for relevant history: Family, diet, social, immunization, etc.	

Contd...

Contd...

Step	***Tick here***
Closing: • Summarize for caregiver and ask if any information is missed • Thank the caregiver for the time	
Summary: • Summarize with name, age of the patient, presenting complaint, and relevant medical history • Make a provisional diagnosis or offer a differential diagnosis	

SECTION

2 Physical Examination

CHAPTER

2.1 Well-Baby Examination

Setting: A day 2 baby is about to be discharged from the hospital. Evaluate the baby.

OBJECTIVE

At the end of examination of an infant at hospital discharge, one should be able to reach following conclusions:

- Is the baby well or sick?
- What is the gestation and weight?
- Are there any physiological findings?
- Are there any clues to pathological conditions?
- Are there any occult anomalies?

CHECKLIST

Step	*Tick here*
Observe the baby for well-being: • Consciousness, color, tone, posture, cry, breathing, activity • *Notes vital parameters:* Temperature, heart rate, respiration (identifies stable, unstable, not well, and in need of further assessment)	
Identify gestation and classify with weight: • Preterm or late preterm or term • Appropriate for gestational age (AGA) or small for gestational age (SGA) or large for gestational age (LGA) • Assess weight, height, and head circumference; use growth chart to plot	
Identify physiological findings: Perform head-to-toe examination	
Identify signs indicating pathology: • Perform occult anomaly search • Ask for pulse oximeter screen • Look for jaundice • Do screening for developmental dysplasia of hip • Check reports of hearing, metabolic screen if done or schedules a visit	
Closing: Thank the caregiver for the time	
Summary: Summarize with name, age of the patient, and key clinical findings	

EXAMINATION FOR WELL-BEING

Look	*Normal*	*Abnormal*
Consciousness	Alert	Drowsy, lethargic, nonresponsive, persistent irritability, asleep
Color	Pink	Pale (anemia, shock), plethora (polycythemia), dusky [cold stress, hypothermia, congenital heart disease (CHD), shock], cyanosis (cold stress, CHD, respiratory failure)
Tone, posture	Active with good tone and responds to pain	Abnormal tone is reflected by posture (frog-legged posture, extended posture) and suggests neurologic compromise
Cry	Lusty cry	Weak, absent, ill sustained or shrill cry
Activity	Symmetric and spontaneous	Decreased, absent, asymmetric and abnormal movements
Temperature	36.5–37.5°C	Cold stress (36–36.5°C), hypothermia (<36°C), core-axillary mismatch (>3°C) or fever (>37.5°C)
Heart rate	Heart rate 120–120 beats/min	To identify rate, rhythm, and monitor the trends
Breathing	Regular, rate 40–60 breaths/min, no audible sounds	Slow <40 or fast >60 breaths/min, Downes score or Silverman–Anderson score, apnea, gasping, chest indrawing, grunt, stridor
Pulse oximeter	>95% after 24 hours of age	Upper limb and lower limb difference of >5, SpO_2 <95% in room air
Note	Rationale	
Anthropometry	Weight, height, and head circumference plotting on growth chart defines growth pattern	
Gestation	Preterm (<34 weeks), post-term, and late preterm (34–37 weeks) are vulnerable population.	

(SpO_2: peripheral oxygen saturation)

HEAD-TO-TOE PHYSICAL EXAMINATION

Assess	*Look for*	*Abnormal*
Skin	Hydration, color	Birthmarks, congenital anomaly, pustules
Head	Size, shape, symmetry Fontanel, sutures	Microcephaly and macrocephaly, molding, craniosynostosis, tense anterior fontanelle, swelling
Eyes	Size, position, slant	White reflex, asymmetry, discharge, redness

Contd...

Contd...

Assess	*Look for*	*Abnormal*
Ears	Shape, size, position	Low set, tags, pits, malformation
Mouth	Shape, position, symmetry	Tongue, gums, tooth swelling
Palate	Anterior/posterior palate	Cleft
Limbs	Symmetry, movements, palmar crease	Polydactyly, syndactyly, clinodactyly, malformation
Umbilicus	Discharge, swelling, redness	Purulent or foul discharge, periumbilical erythema, hernia
Genitalia	*Boys*: penile size, urethral opening, scrotal symmetry, rugosity, testis in scrotum *Girls*: Labia majora–minora, clitoris, urethra–vagina	Penis <1 cm, chordee, hypospadias, epispadias, absent scrotal rugosity, empty scrotum, asymmetric scrotum hymenal tags, discharge per urethra–vagina
Back—spine	Spine curvature	Defect, tufts of hair
Hips	Thigh crease symmetry, Barlow–Otolarni maneuver	Asymmetry, leg shortening
Urine/stool	Color, odor, frequency	High-colored urine, clay stools, red stools

Note	*Comment*
Physiological signs	Erythema toxicum, jaundice, caput, Epstein's pearl, breast fullness, peeling of skin, acne, vaginal discharge, capillary hemangioma, Mongolian spots, meconium staining of cord
Occult congenital anomalies	Isolated cleft palate, cataract, anogenital anomalies, spinal defects and absent femoral pulses need to be specifically looked at
Danger signs	• Grunt, cyanosis, worsening sensorium, apnea, jaundice up to palms and soles, weak or absent cry, abnormal or asymmetric movements • To identify life-threatening events and consider urgent transfer/interventions

SUMMARIZE

A male baby of Nisha, term, AGA, 36 hours of birth has birth weight of 2.7 kg. His vital signs are stable, with physiological findings such as erythema toxicum, caput succedaneum, and Mongolian spots. There are no hidden anomalies or pathological signs, indicating a healthy, full-term newborn. He is scheduled for a newborn screening [thyroid stimulating hormone (TSH), expanded newborn screening (ENBS)] and hearing evaluation 2 days later.

CHAPTER 2.2

Assessment of Breastfeeding

CHECKLIST

Step	*Tick here*
Examine the breast for flat nipple/inverted nipple/engorgement/ pain/sore nipples or mastitis in the breast after informing the informant	
Examine the neonate for evidence of dehydration (assess for weight, sunken fontanel, pallor, lethargy and overall activity)	
Examine for cardinal points of positioning **(Fig. 1)**: • Head in line with the body • Whole body well-supported • Neonate turned toward the mother • Neonate's abdomen touching the mother's abdomen	
Examine for cardinal points of attachment **(Figs. 2A and B)**: • More areola visible above the neonate's mouth than below it • Neonate's mouth is wide open • Neonate's lower lip is turn outward • Neonate's chin is touching the mother's breast	

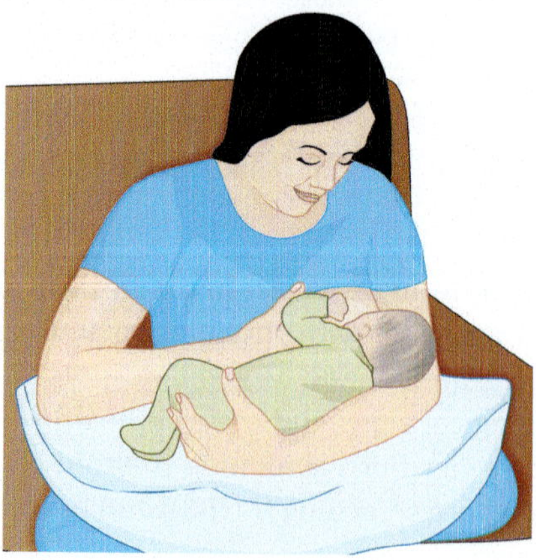

Fig. 1: Cradle hold.

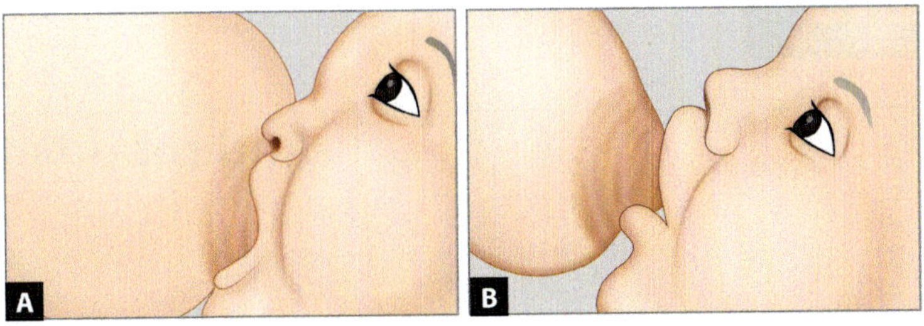

Figs. 2A and B: (A) A baby well attached to his mother's breast; (B) A baby poorly attached to his mother's breast.

CHAPTER 2.3

Anthropometry

MEASUREMENT OF LENGTH

Equipment: Infantometer, cloth for covering the base, and mother or assistant.

Procedure

Checklist	*Tick here*
Ask the assistant to help with measurement and to comfort the baby	
Cover the length board with a thin cloth or soft paper	
Explain to the assistant where to stand when placing the baby on length board, i.e., opposite to you, on the side of the length board away from the tape	
Lay the baby on his back with his head against the fixed headboard, compressing the hair	
Position the head so that an imaginary vertical line from the ear canal to the lower border of the eye socket is perpendicular to the board (the baby's eyes should be looking straight up)	
Ask the assistant to hold the head in this position	
Check that the infant lies straight along the board and does not change position. Shoulders should touch the board, and the spine should not be arched	
Hold down the infant's legs with one hand and move the footboard with the other. Apply gentle pressure to the knees to straighten the legs as far as they can go without causing injury	
While holding the knees, pull the footboard against the infant's feet. The soles of the feet should be flat against the footboard, toes pointing upward	
Read the measurement and record the infant's length in centimeters to the last *completed* 0.1 cm in the notes of the growth record. This is the last line that you can actually see (0.1 cm = 1 mm)	

Note:

- If an infant is extremely agitated and both legs cannot be held in position, measure with one leg in position.
- If the infant bends the toes and prevents the footboard from touching the soles, scratch the soles slightly and slide in the footboard quickly when the infant straightens the toes.

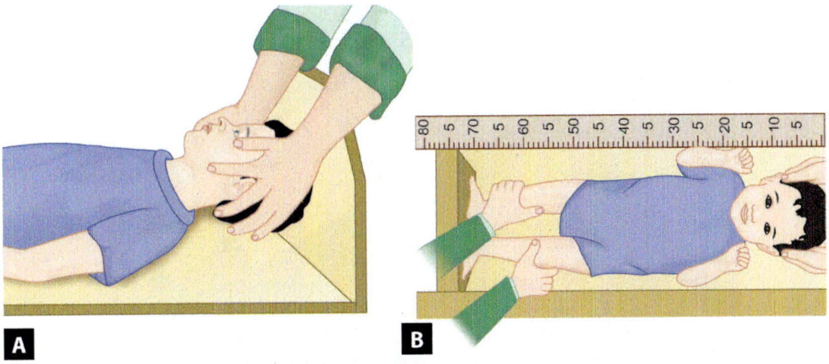

Figs. 1A and B: Measurement of length.

- Record the length on the growth chart and present as length in centiles **(Figs. 1A and B)**.

MEASUREMENT OF WEIGHT

Equipment: Digital weighing scale; it is accurate and has a precision of weighing 0.01 kg or 10 g. It has an option of zeroing.

Procedure

Checklist	*Tick here*
Ask the assistant to assist you in weighing the baby	
Ensure a sterile baby towel is placed on the pan	
Ensure zeroing of the machine before placing the baby	
Weight the baby naked	
Note the value once the baby is relatively calm. Wait for the fluctuations to settle down	
Record the weight on the growth chart and present as weight in centiles	

MEASUREMENT OF THE HEAD CIRCUMFERENCE

Equipment: A flexible and nonstretchable tape **(Fig. 2)**.

Procedure

Checklist	*Tick here*
Ask the mother to assist you by making the baby comfortable	
Position the tape just above the eyebrows, above the ears, and around the biggest part of the back of the head	
Pull the tape snugly to compress the hair	
The overlapping of the tape should be done on the lateral aspect of the head (avoid the curves), to get accurate value	
Read the nearest 0.1 cm, by cross tape technique	
Plot the head circumference on the growth curve and present in centiles	

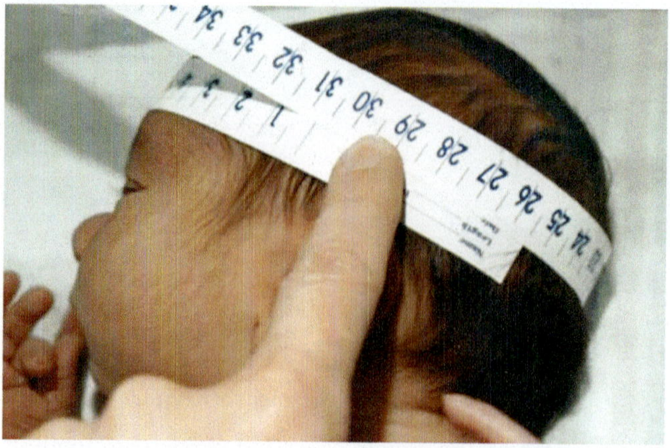

Fig. 2: Measurement of head circumference.

CHAPTER

2.4 Capillary Refill Time

INTRODUCTION

Capillary refill time (CRT) is time taken for color to return to an external capillary bed after pressure is applied to cause blanching **(Figs. 1A and B)**.

PROCEDURE

Checklist	*Tick here*
Ensure warmth	
Expose the chest of the infant	
Use thumb or finger and press on the sternum for 5 seconds	
Remove the thumb/finger and see the time taken for blanched area to become pink again	

Note:

- The mnemonic used is "one in one thousand, two in one thousand, three in one thousand, four in one thousand, five in one thousand".
- The normal CRT is <3 seconds.

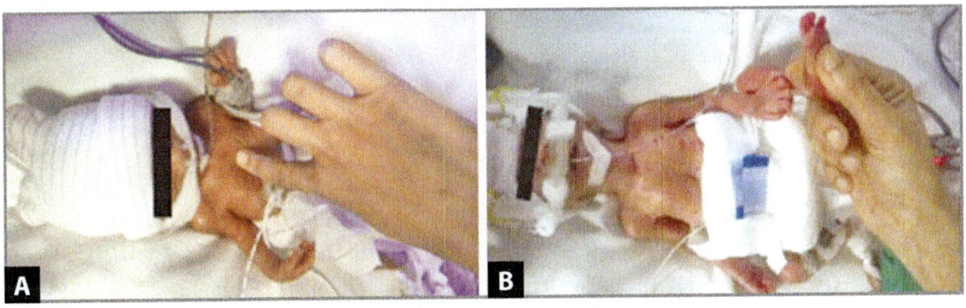

Figs. 1A and B: Capillary refill time.

CHAPTER 2.5

Fontanel Examination

Setting: A day 5 baby is admitted for irritability to the hospital. Evaluate the baby's fontanel.

OBJECTIVE

At the end of examination in an irritable infant for fontanel, one should be able to reach following conclusions:

- Is the anterior fontanel and posterior fontanel palpable?
- What is the size, pulsatility of the fontanel?
- Is it normal or abnormal?

CHECKLIST

Step	*Tick here*
Fontanel evaluation: • Ensure the baby is in supine position in quiet state • Lift the head slightly from the bed • Palpate the anterior fontanel (AF) at the junction of coronal and sagittal suture. Note the dimension and pulsatility • Palpate the posterior fontanel (PF) at the junction of lambdoidal and sagittal suture. Note the dimensions • Auscultate over the AF for any bruit	

Note:

- *Pulsatility:* Normal fontanel is pulsatile. Absence of pulsations suggest raised intracranial pressure.
- *Size:* Note the maximum anteroposterior diameter (AP) and transverse diameter (T) to calculate the fontanel size = (AP + T)/2
- *Contour:* Normally the fontanel is at soft, level, and flat.
- A bulging or sunken fontanel is abnormal.
- Auscultate for bruit. It is heard with arteriovenous (AV) malformation.

CHAPTER 2.6

Palmar Grasp

CHECKLIST

Steps	Tick here
• Ensure the infant is awake and alert • Ensure baby is lying in supine position on a flat comfortable surface/ mother's lap with head in midline • Ensure that dorsum of hands (of baby) is not touching the bed/towel or any other object • Place little finger (preferably)/index finger along ulnar aspect of baby's palm and applies pressure gently onto palm • *Note for appropriate response:* Flexion of all fingers around the examiner's finger and closure of hand • Apply mild traction as if trying to pull finger away from baby's palm • Note for increasing tightening of baby's grip and clinging, one may also be able to gently lift a term baby off the couch with this grip itself • Gently remove the finger from baby's grip—if not able to remove, one can gently stimulate the dorsum of same hand (which should elicit opening of hands) • Repeat the same process on the other side	

SUMMARIZE (WHEN ASKED)

- Term/preterm
- Postmenstrual age/corrected age
- State or sensorium of baby
- Response—optimal/not optimal, symmetric/asymmetric

Note:

- *Age of appearance:* noted in utero around 16 weeks, may be elicited in a preterm by 25 weeks PMA
- *Age of disappearance:* Easily elicited in the first 3 months of life (corrected age if preterm), usually disappears by 6 months. Replaced by voluntary hand movements
- Note whether there are any attachments on the hands [peripheral oxygen saturation (SpO_2) probe, intravenous cannula] that can interfere with/ affect response.

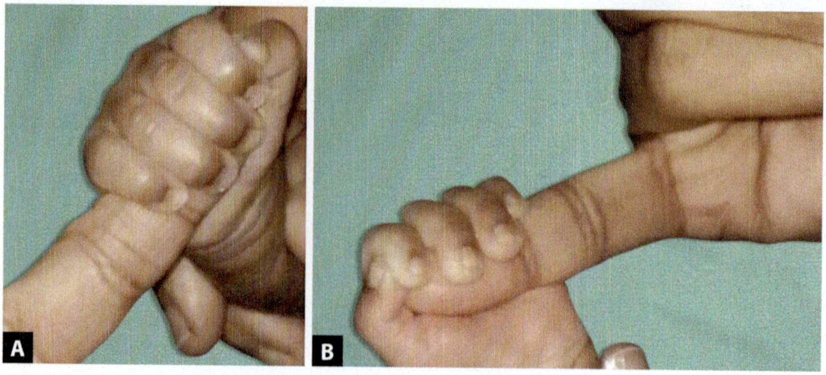

Figs. 1A and B: Palmar grasp reflex.

WHAT IS AN ABNORMAL RESPONSE?

- If the reflex is not elicited or weak during the age when it normally should be present:
  - Usually, lower motor neuron lesions like root, plexus, nerve, spinal cord injury
  - Generalized neonatal encephalopathy
  - May not be elicited in evolving athetoid cerebral palsy
- If the reflex is exaggerated or persists beyond the age of normal disappearance:
  - Spastic cerebral palsy
- Persistence may lead to poor handwriting, poor manual dexterity, or impairment of fine motor skills **(Figs. 1A and B)**.

CHAPTER 2.7

Plantar Grasp

CHECKLIST

Steps	*Tick here*
• Ensure the baby is awake and alert • Ensure baby is lying in supine position on flat surface with head in midline • Place thumb on the sole of the foot below the toes and apply gentle pressure • Note appropriate response—flexion of all toes **(Fig. 1)** • Repeat on other side	

SUMMARIZE (WHEN ASKED)

- Term/preterm
- Postmenstrual age (PMA)/corrected age
- State or sensorium of baby
- Response—optimal/not optimal, symmetric/asymmetric

NEED TO KNOW

- *Age of appearance:* Elicited in preterm from 25 weeks PMA
- *Age of disappearance:* Easily elicited in the first 6 months of life (corrected age if preterm), usually disappears by 12 months; disappearance is significantly related to commencement of standing.
- Note whether there are any attachments on the feet [peripheral oxygen saturation (SpO_2) probe, intravenous cannula] that can interfere with/affect response.

WHAT IS AN ABNORMAL RESPONSE?

If the reflex is not elicited or weak during the age when it normally should be present, it is an abnormal response.

- Usually, lower motor neuron lesions like root, plexus, nerve, and spinal cord injury
- Generalized neonatal encephalopathy
- May not be elicited in evolving spastic cerebral palsy.

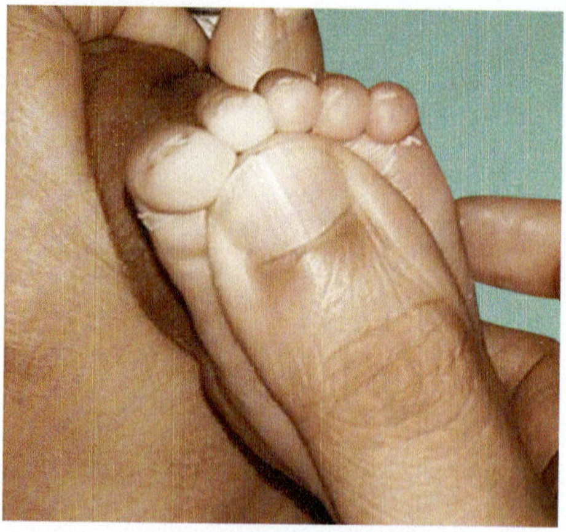

Fig. 1: Plantar grasp reflex.

A weak or reduced plantar response has been shown to be a sensitive indicator of later development of spasticity. The side of abnormal response correlates well with the laterality of later motor abnormalities like in spastic hemiplegia.

If the reflex is exaggerated or persists beyond the age of normal disappearance, then it is athetoid cerebral palsy.

Persistence may lead to awkwardness while walking, poor balance, and problems with sports requiring balance and coordination while running.

CHAPTER 2.8

Moro's Reflex

CHECKLIST

Step	*Tick here*
Ensure the baby is alert and in quiet state	
Ensure head is in midline	
Head drop method: The infant is held suspended in a symmetrical supine position with one of the examiner's hands behind the chest and the other supporting the head, allow the head to be dropped back a few cm	
Note: • Abduction of the upper limbs (spreading out arms) • Opening of the fist • Crying • Adduction of the upper limbs (unspreading the arms) • The reflex is complete and symmetrical on both the sides	

Note:

- This primitive reflex emerges at 8–9 weeks in utero, is present at birth, and normally disappears after 3 or 4 months.
- An absent reflex is seen in upper motor neuron lesions, e.g., severe perinatal asphyxia, intracranial hemorrhage, infection, brain malformation, general muscular weakness of any cause, and cerebral palsy (CP) of the spastic type.
- An asymmetric Moro is most often seen with local cause, e.g., damage to peripheral nerve (brachial plexus lesion, cervical cord lesion) or fracture bone (clavicle).
- Postnatal persistence occurs in infants with severe neurological defects.
- An exaggerated response may also be detected in infants with a severe bilateral intrauterine lesion (e.g., hydranencephaly).
- Ensure that both the subject's hands are open at the moment of elicitation of the reflex so as not to provoke an asymmetrical response.
- If the baby is crying, allow the baby to quiet down before eliciting the response.

CHAPTER 2.9

Asymmetric Tonic Neck Reflex

CHECKLIST

Step	*Tick here*
Ensure the baby is in a quiet but alert state	
Ensure the baby is in supine position with head in midline to start with	
Turn the head of the baby gently so that the face looks toward any one side	
Note the appropriate response: The arms and legs on the side of the face extend; and the other side limbs flex (classical fencing posture)	
Repeat by turning the head to another side and note the response	

Note:

- Ensure there are no attachments on the hands [peripheral oxygen saturation (SpO_2) probe, intravenous cannula] that can interfere with/ affect response.
- If baby turns head spontaneously to any side—can note for appropriate response without touching the baby.
- *Age of appearance:* 18 weeks of gestation (noted in utero)
- *Age of disappearance:* The reflex should be inhibited 4–6 months of age (corrected age if preterm) in the awake state, beyond which persistence is considered abnormal.

DIFFERENTIALS FOR NONOPTIMAL RESPONSE

- Decreased/no response can be normal (the reflex is best observed rather than elicited)
- Depressed sensorium due to various conditions leading to neonatal encephalopathy can lead to decreased response.
- Asymmetric tonic neck reflex (ATNR) is required in early infancy to establish visual-motor (hand-eye) coordination.
- A retained ATNR is associated with abnormalities in motor, academic, and social development domains. Infants and children are noted to have:
    - Poor gross motor coordination and balance; turning to any side might lead to change in ipsilateral limb tone and loss of balance.
    - Difficulty with visual tracking, activities that need crossing the midline like writing across a page from left to right or reading a line and following text
    - Poor eye-hand coordination as in school learning and sports

CHAPTER 2.10

Developmental Dysplasia of Hip

CHECKLIST

Step	Tick here
Inspection: • Undress the baby to examine the spine and hip • Grossly note general health status • *Look for dysmorphic features:* Teratological developmental dysplasia of hip accompanies arthrogryposis and spinal dysraphism • Inspect the back for spina bifida or meningocele	

Lower limb examination:
• *Inspect for limb length discrepancy (Galeazzi sign):*
  – Flex lower limbs at knees
  – Place heels together with soles of feet flat on bed
  – Make sure pelvis is square and look at level of knees. Inequality in the height of the knees is a positive Galeazzi sign
• Inspect thigh creases, groin crease, and gluteal folds by holding up the child as well as placing the child prone
• Note any asymmetry on ventral/dorsal surfaces	

Test abduction: • Flex hips to right angle and test range of abduction • Dislocated hip will be tighter and have restriction of movement	

Specific test:
• *Barlow test*: Provocative dislocation of a reduced hip
  – It is positive when an enlocated (suggest unstable) hip can be dislocated or subluxated. Each hip should be examined separately. The pelvis should be stabilized by holding the contralateral hip.
  – Flex lower limb at knee and hip
  – Adduct the baby's hip, gently applying a downward force by pushing the knee gently posteriorly (i.e., downward)
  – Normally, there is a small amount of movement
  – But in abnormal hip, the force will subluxate/dislocate the joint and a "clunk" will be felt
• *Ortolani test*: Reduction maneuver of a dislocated hip.
  – It is positive when a dislocated hip is relocated
  – Place thumbs medially and index finger high on posterolateral aspect of thigh (behind greater trochanter)	

Contd…

Contd…

Step	*Tick here*
– Hips flexed to 90° and gently abducted, simultaneously exerting upward pressure through the greater trochanter – Normally, it is a easy abduction – But in dislocated hip, the force will relocate the head in the acetabulum at the joint and a "clunk" will be felt • *Klisic's test*: – Line drawn from greater trochanter to anterior superior iliac spine (ASIS) should continue medially – If line pass toward the umbilicus—hip is normal – If line passes below umbilicus—hip is dislocated	
Associated disorders: • Plagiocephaly • Torticollis • Calcaneovalgus foot • Metatarsus adductus	

CHAPTER

2.11 New Ballard Score

INTRODUCTION

Ask the learner to assess the gestation of a preterm baby by New Ballard Score (NBS) **(Table 1)**. Baby should be preterm, and gestation should be 28–34 weeks. Baby should be hemodynamically stable, and age should be <96 hours (or less desirably <7 days). Provide following chart and assess how gestation is assessed.

- Explain to the mother or parent the process.
- Perform hand hygiene.
- *Examine as per chart (12 parameters)*:
  - Complete all points.
  - Assess each parameter by correct method.
- Provide value of assessed gestation.

TABLE 1: New Ballard Score.

Neuromuscular maturity

Score	–1	0	1	2	3	4	5
Posture							
Square window (wrist)	>90°	90°	60°	45°	30°	0°	
Arm recoil		180°	140°–180°	110°–140°	90°–110°	<90°	
Popliteal angle	180°	160°	140°	120°	100°	90°	<90°
Scarf sign							
Heel to ear							

Contd...

Contd...

Physical maturity								
Skin	Sticky, friable, transparent	Gelatinous, red, translucent	Smooth, pink; visible veins	Superficial peeling and/or rash; few veins	Cracking, pale areas; rare veins	Parchment, deep cracking; no vessels	Leathery, cracked, wrinkled	
Lanugo	None	Sparse	Abundant	Thinning	Bald areas	Mostly bad	Maturity rating	
Plantar surface	Heel—100 40–50 mm: −1 <40 mm: −2	>50 mm, no crease	Faint red marks	Anterior transverse crease only	Crease anterior 2/3	Creases over entire sole	Score −10 −5	Weeks 20 22
Breast	Imperceptible	Barely perceptible	Flat areola, no bud	Stippled areola, 1–2 mm bud	Raised areola. 3–4 mm bud	Full areola, 5–10 mm bud	0 5	24 26
Eye/Ear	Lids fused loosely: −1, tightly −2	Lids open; pinna flat; stays folded	Slightly curved pinna; soft slow recoil	Well-curved pinna; soft but ready recoil	Raised areola, 3–4 mm bud	Testes pendulous, deep rugae	10 15 20 25	28 30 32 34
Genitals (male)	Scrotum flat, smooth	Scrotum empty, faint, rugae	Testes in upper canal, rare rugae	Testes descending, few rugae	Testes down good rugae	Testes pendulous deep rugae	30 35 40	36 38 40
Genitals (female)	Clitoris prominent, labia flat	Clitoris prominent, small labia minora	Clitoris prominent, enlarging minora	Majora and minora equally prominent	Majora large, minora small	Majora cover clitoris and minora	45 50	42 44

Note:

- If the assessed gestation is >2 weeks more or less than reported, assessed gestation is preferred.
- Gestation can be assessed for infants from 20 to 44 weeks.
- NBS can be done even in sick newborns.
- In the first 12 hours after birth, oxytocin affects the joint laxity.
- In intrauterine growth restriction (IUGR), individual components such as breast bud, skin creases, posture, and arm recoil are affected.

CHAPTER 2.12

Tone Assessment

ASSESS THE TONE OF THE HAMSTRING MUSCLES

Checklist	*Tick here*
• Ensure the newborn is in a quiet and alert state • Elicit tone in one leg at a time • Ensure that the pelvis is not lifted off the bed • With the infant lying supine, remove the diaper • The thigh is placed gently on the baby's abdomen with the knee fully flexed. Wait until the infant stops kicking actively before extending the leg • Gently grasp the foot at the sides with one hand while supporting the side of the thigh with the other. Extend the leg until a definite resistance to extension is appreciated • Note the angle between the thigh and the leg. It is typically about 90° • Compare response of both the legs	

Note:

- Extension of the leg beyond 90°–120° would be seen in hypotonia.
- The prenatal frank breech position will interfere with this maneuver for the first 24–48 hours **(Fig. 1)**.

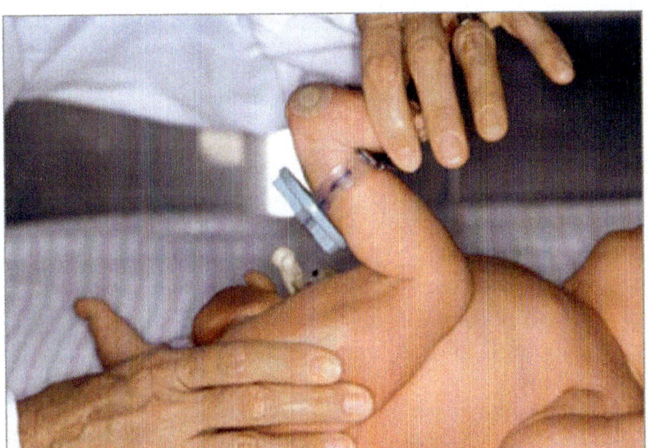

Popliteal angle	180°	160°	140°	120°	100°	90°	<90°

Fig. 1: Popliteal angle measurement.

HEEL-TO-EAR EXAMINATION

Checklist	*Tick here*
• Ensure the infant is quiet • The infant is placed supine • Support the infant's thigh laterally alongside the body with the palm of one hand. The other hand grasps the infant's foot at the sides to pull it toward the ipsilateral ear • Note the location of the heel where significant resistance is appreciated. Observe the distance between feet and head • Keep the pelvis flat on the bed • Elicit on one leg at a time	

Note: The heel in a normal baby would only come to midchest. If the foot can be drawn to the ear, then there is hypotonia **(Fig. 2)**.

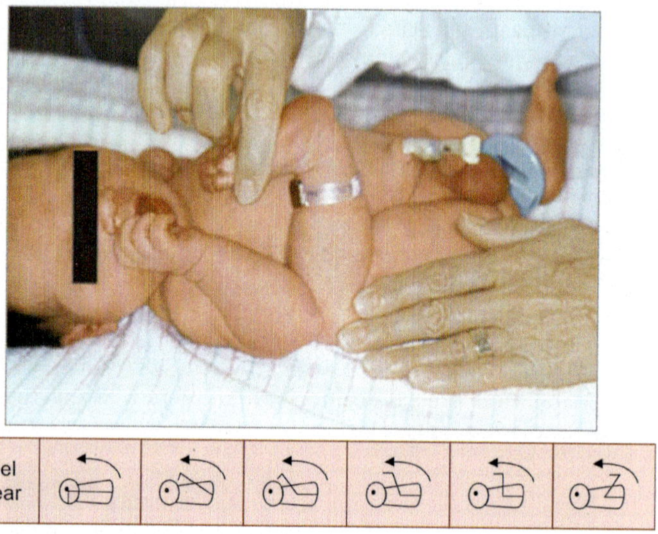

Fig. 2: Heel-to-ear examination.

SCARF SIGN

Checklist	*Tick here*
• Ensure the infant is in supine position, alert but in a quiet state • Hold the infant's hand and try to bring it around the neck and as posteriorly as possible over the opposite shoulder • The other hand supports the baby's chest and the thumb of is placed on the infant's elbow • The point on the chest to which the elbow moves easily prior to significant resistance is noted **(Fig. 3)**	

Note: The hand should not go past the shoulder and the elbow should not cross the midline in term infants.

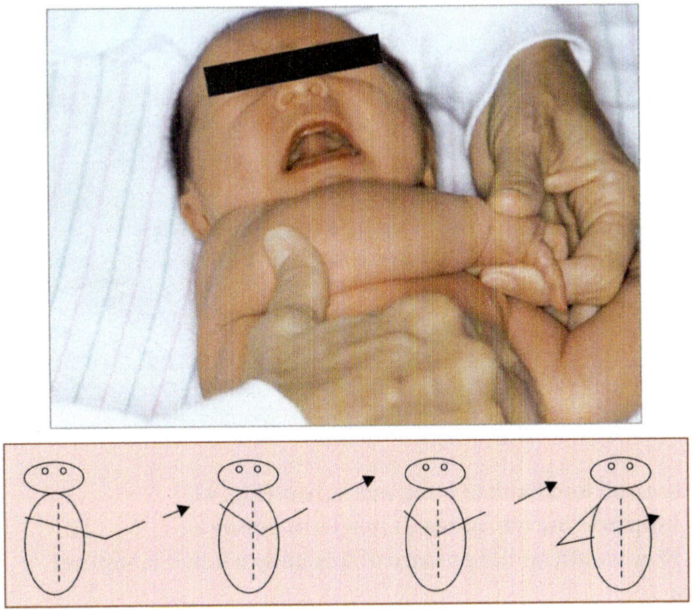

Fig. 3: Scarf sign.

ASSESSMENT OF SHOULDER TONE

Focused clinical examination:

1. **How to assess shoulder tone in newborn?**

   Ans: The assessment of shoulder tone in newborns includes:
   - Posture
   - *Passive tone:* Ensure head in midline for all maneuvers to avoid effect of asymmetrical tonic neck reflex (ATNR).
   - Scarf sign
   - Forearm recoil
   - *Active tone:* Raise to sit and back to lying maneuver.
   - Horizontal suspension
   - Vertical suspension
   - *Primitive reflexes:* Finger grasp and response to traction

2. **What are the normal parameters for shoulder tone evaluation?**

Finding	*<32 weeks*	*34 weeks*	*36 weeks*	*Normal term*
Scarf sign				
Forearm recoil				
Raise to sit				
Back to lying				

Ans:

Finding	*<32 weeks*	*34 weeks*	*36 weeks*	*Normal term*
Scarf sign	Arm encircles neck at 28 weeks	Elbow largely passes midline	Elbow slightly passes midline	Elbow does not cross midline
Forearm recoil	Extension	Weak	Present	Strong
Raise to sit	No head movement forwards	Head rolls on shoulder	Head briskly passes in axis	Perfect minimal lag
Back to lying	No head movement backwards	Head passes briskly in axis	Powerful movement backwards	Perfect minimal lag

3. **Raise to sit and back to lying maneuver (Fig. 4).**
   a. **Interpret the above result in a term neonate.**
   b. **How would be the posture of this baby when it is supine?**

   Ans:
   a. *Hypertonia of neck extensors*: Raise to sit—head does not pass the axis nor move forward at end of maneuver. Back to lying movement is too good.
   b. *Retrocollis*: Neck extended, head to one side

   Or

   Opisthotonus: Arching of whole-body axis with neck and spine extensor hypertonia.

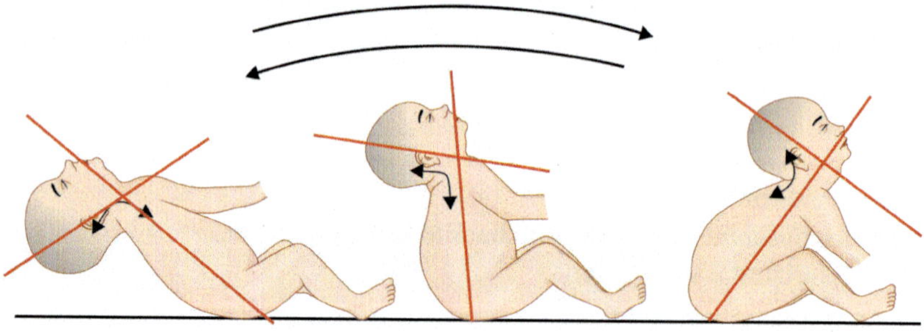

Fig. 4: Assessment of shoulder tone.

4. **What would you look for in the general examination of a newborn baby with abnormal shoulder tone evaluation in each of the following?**
   a. Eyes
   b. Skin
   c. Head
   d. Face
   e. Mouth

f. Chest
g. Joints
h. Spine

Ans:

a. *Eyes:* Hypertonia elevator palpebrae superioris, nystagmus, fixation and tracking movements, acoustic blink.
b. *Skin:* Neurocutaneous markers.
c. *Head:* Anterior fontanels, sutures—overriding, squamous suture.
d. *Face:* Dysmorphic features (Downs, Prader Wili)
e. *Examination of mouth and tongue:*
   i. Palate—high arched (abnormal motor function of fetal tongue)
   ii. Fasciculations at rest in periphery of tongue (Werdnig-Hoffmann)
f. *Chest movements:* Indrawing of sternum (Werd-Hoffmann).
g. *Joints:* Arthrogryposis (suggests antenatal neuromuscular etiology)
h. *Spine:* Dysraphism

5. **What is the clinical significance of abnormal shoulder tone?**

Ans: The clinical significance of abnormal shoulder tone includes:

a. Trunk and neck abnormalities
b. Increased or decreased shoulder tone delays midline hand play, reach and transfer
c. Increased shoulder tone interferes with hand to mouth pattern

CHAPTER

2.13

Hammersmith Neonatal Neurological Examination

CHECKLIST

Step	*Tick here*
Introduce to the family the purpose of testing:	
1. *Pretesting:* a. Know the right age to test the baby b. *Hammersmith neonatal neurological examination (HNNE)* is best tested at 2 weeks of age in term babies and estimated term age [40 weeks post-menstrual age (PMA)] in preterm babies c. Baby should be awake and alert, not hungry and crying d. Center the baby's head—ask mother to hold gently	
2. *Observe tone and posture:* a. Posture of baby in alert resting state—greater importance given to match the *lower limb posture* with picture on the chart. Watch for asymmetry in tone and posture (head should be in midline) b. Upper limb—traction—hold the wrist and not the palm, look and feel tone at elbow c. Upper limb—arm recoil d. Lower limb traction—hold the ankle and not the foot, look and feel tone at knee e. Popliteal angle—baby on bed, flex the thighs on to the abdomen, pelvis in contact with bed. Use index fingers to deflex the knee (popliteal) joint. Measure angle between leg and bed. Ensure head in midline before inferring asymmetry. Popliteal angle tightness is best interpreted in relation to leg traction (tone patterns—item i). f. Trunk in ventral suspension—look for trunk tone and limb tone g. Head lag in pull to sit h. Head control—flexors and extensors—place the baby is sitting posture, encircle the chest with your palm and fingers. Allow the head to fall forward gently (to test extensors) and watch for head being lifted transiently to straight position. Repeat the test with head allowed to fall backward gently (to test flexors). Best evaluated by comparing the flexors and extensors (tone patterns—item i). Well-developed extensors in relation to flexors point to possibly evolving cerebral palsy i. Evaluate tone patterns—real difference in tone inferred if one column difference is found between compared items: a. Upper—lower limb b. Popliteal—leg traction c. Head control flexor—extensor	

Contd...

Contd...

Step	*Tick here*
3. *Movements:* a. *Quantity and quality:* Abnormal writhing, cramped, and stereotyped movements b. *Abnormal movements:* Tremors, startle, and spontaneous abnormal movements that are persistent.	
4. *Abnormal patterns:* a. Cortical thumb, and index finger opposed b. Spontaneous upgoing big toe, flexed toes of foot	
5. *Reflexes:* a. Moro's reflex b. Palmar grasp c. Plantar grasp d. Sucking reflex e. Deep tendon reflexes f. Stepping and placing reflexes	
6. *Orientation*: a. Arousability and consolability—Baby's change in behavior is noted as examiner uncovers the baby. Most babies will be easy to arouse and start crying (baby will appear difficult to arouse if baby just had a feed). If baby is difficult to calm by patting gently or cuddling, this may suggest abnormal behavior (baby will appear difficult to console if baby is hungry) b. Visual orientation—slowly dangling red ball or ring, or human face is presented at a distance about 18 inches (distance from breast to mother's face when baby is breastfed) c. Auditory orientation—sound introduced from behind (not in line of vision)—distance about 10–15 cm from ear (distance from breast to mother's face when baby is breastfed)	
7. Examine head size, shape, and spine	
8. Summarize examination findings	

Note:

- HNNE is a comprehensive evaluation of functioning of the nervous system. Any deviation from "optimal", i.e., from what is common to babies, will need further evaluation.
- *Testing*:
  - *Optimal:* Noted in up to 90% of healthy newborns
  - *Suboptimal:* Found in <10% babies
    - Single, transient signs have no clinical relevance. Persistence of signs over time and deviation from optimal in two or more signs warrant detail evaluation.

Clinical value:

- As a screening tool—the suboptimal neuroposture or behavior are in "black" boxes, they need to be re-evaluated for persistence of signs.

- As a research tool—each evaluated item can be converted into scores. If 90% babies demonstrate the sign, it is considered as optimal. Items are scored as suboptimal or not optimal if only 10% or less of babies demonstrate the sign.

Strengths of HNNE:
- Comprehensive examination of all domains of nervous system
- Easy to do, even for non-neurologist
- Takes only 10–15 minutes to complete
- Good interobserver reliability
- Allows evaluation for persistence of signs and evolution of signs
- Validated against magnetic resonance imaging (MRI) in prediction of outcomes

When is HNNE inaccurate?
- Baby on sedatives or antiepileptic drugs
- Isolated deviant signs have limited value. Deviation of one/two signs is found in one-third of the healthy population.

CHAPTER 2.14

Denver Developmental Screening

CHECKLIST

Step	Tick here
Pretest preparation: • Ensure environment is child friendly • Child is well • Denver Developmental Screening Test II (DDST-II) kit and form available, kept ready out of sight of child • Calculate corrected age • Draw corrected age line on the chart • Allay parental anxiety and reassure	
Administering DDST-II: • Do in presence of parents/caregiver • Start administering items to the left of the line in the chart in each sector and continue to the right • Administer items needing less active participation first like report, personal social, then fine motor-adaptive, language, and lastly gross motor items • In each sector, administer at least three items to the left of the line and every item intersected by the age line • Testing may be flexible • Rate test behavior after completion of the test • Fill chart • Explain results to parents and action plan	
Interpret: • As normal, suspect or untestable • Provide score	

Fill the table based on a DDST-II chart and give remarks.

Classification	Scores	Action
Normal		
Suspect		
Untestable		

Answer:

Classification	*Scores*	*Action*
Normal	No delay ± maximum 1 caution	Routine follow-up
Suspect	2 or more caution and 1 or more delays	• Rescreen in 1–2 weeks • If retest suspect, do DASII and neuromotor evaluation • Start early intervention
Untestable	Refusal in 1 or more item to left of line or refusal in 1 item in line in shaded area.	• Rescreen in 1–2 weeks • If retest untestable or suspect, do DASII and neuromotor evaluation • Start early intervention

(DASII: Developmental Assessment Scale for Indian Infants)

CHAPTER 2.15

Jaundice

Setting: This day 3 baby is brought by parents for yellowish discoloration of the body. Examine the baby for jaundice.

OBJECTIVE

At the end of examination in an infant with jaundice, one should be able to reach following conclusions:

- Is jaundice present? Is it direct or indirect?
- What is the extent and severity of jaundice?
- Are there any clues to pathological jaundice?
- Are there any complications due to jaundice?
- What is the probable underlying cause?

CHECKLIST

Step	*Tick here*
• *Identify jaundice and the type of jaundice*: – Examine the baby naked in daylight – Look for yellowness over the sclera, face, trunk, abdomen, legs and hands, palms and soles. – Check for color and staining of urine and stool color. – Ask for age in hours of the jaundice baby.	
• *Identify the extent of jaundice:* Apply digital pressure over forehead, sternum, abdomen, thigh, palms, and soles to look for yellowish discoloration	
• *Identify severity of jaundice*: – Observe sensorium, posture, tone, cry, and activity. – Check for sucking reflex, Moro reflex – Check for setting sun sign, shrill or weak cry, and tone abnormality (opisthotonus, dystonia, hypo- or hypertonia)	
• *Identify clues to pathological jaundice*: – *Sick baby:* Unstable vital parameters, respiratory or circulatory insufficiency – *Gestation:* Late Preterm, preterm infant – *Weight:* Appropriate for gestational age (AGA), small for gestational age (SGA), large for gestational age (LGA), weight loss >7%	

Contd...

Contd...

Step	Tick here
– *Lactational adequacy:* Check birth weight and current weight, ask for maternal fullness of breasts, maternal concerns, and enquire for the color, frequency of urine and stool of the baby – *Infection:* Thermal instability, fast breathing, grunt, poor activity, irritability, pustules, foul smell, umbilical discharge, bleeding tendency, rash, abnormal movements – *Hemolysis:* Pallor, splenomegaly – *Asphyxia:* Caput, sensorium, irritability, jitteriness, pupillary reaction, seizures – *Others:* Cephalhematoma, subgaleal hemorrhage, polycythemia – *Ask for aggravating factors:* Hypoxia, hypoglycemia, acidosis, hypercarbia	
• *Closing:* Thank the caregiver for the time	
• *Summary:* – Summarize with name, age of the patient, key clinical findings – Make a provisional diagnosis or offer a differential diagnosis	

CONCLUSION

A 74 hours, boy of Radha, near-term gestation, AGA, well baby, with jaundice up to thighs, with >10% weight loss with no features of asphyxia, infection, or hemolysis, and with no abnormality of tone, posture, and activity suggests indirect hyperbilirubinemia with no clinical evidence of bilirubin encephalopathy most probably due to inadequate feeding jaundice.

CHAPTER 2.16

Bilirubin Encephalopathy

Setting: This day 3 baby is admitted for severe jaundice and is under phototherapy. You are to assess for evidence of bilirubin encephalopathy.

OBJECTIVE

At the end of examination of an infant with jaundice under phototherapy, one should be able to reach following conclusions:

- Know how to perform Bilirubin-Induced Neurological Dysfunction (BIND) score.
- Designate the score by using BIND score.
- Know the clinical implications of scoring.

CHECKLIST

Step	*Tick here*
• *Identify component of BIND score:* Observe mental status, tone, cry and sunset sign	
• *Assessment of mental status:* Look for alertness, sleepy but arousable, lethargy, irritability, poor suck or nonresponsiveness	
• *Assessment of muscle tone:* – Note the posture, quality, and symmetry of the movements – Observe the posture at rest, which reflects the active tone and assess the righting reactions of lower extremities and trunk, and righting of head on trunk – For passive tone perform the horizontal and vertical suspension	
• *Assessment of cry:* – Flick the baby soles for crying – Note whether the cry is normal, high-pitched, shrill, weak or absent	
• *Identify BIND score:* Give a score of 0, 1, 2, and 3 for assessment of mental status, tone and cry	
• Interpret BIND score	
• Identify plan of action	

BIND SCORE

Score	*Mental status*	*Tone*	*Cry*
0	Normal	Normal	Normal
1	Sleepy, arousable	Mild hypotonia	High-pitched
2	Lethargy, Irritable	Moderate hypotonia or hypertonia	Shrill
3	Seizures, apnea, coma	Opisthotonus, retrocollis, bicycling	Inconsolable, weak or absent

INTERPRETING BIND SCORE

BIND score	*Action*	*Outcome*
0–3	Intensive phototherapy (PT) and early exchange if signs persist after PT and supportive care	Good
4–6	Intensive PT and exchange transfusion if total serum bilirubin (TSB) in exchange zone	Fairly reversible
>7	Exchange transfusion	Guarded, irreversible

Prediction of 3- to 5-month neurodevelopmental outcomes from signs of *acute bilirubin toxicity*:

BIND score ≥4—specificity (87.3%), sensitivity (97.4%)

CHAPTER

2.17

Poor Weight Gain

Setting: This day 16 baby is brought by parents for concerns of poor weight gain. Examine the baby to identify cause of poor weight gain.

OBJECTIVE

At the end of examination in an infant with suspected weight gain, one should be able to reach following conclusions:

- Identify weight pattern as normal or abnormal.
- Perform lactation adequacy check.
- Identify clinical clues to poor weight gain.

CHECKLIST

Step	*Tick here*
• *Identify weight pattern:* – Note the birth weight and current weight – Interpret weight with gestation and postnatal age – Plot weight on growth chart	
• *Perform lactation adequacy check:* – Check diaper. Note the color and frequency of urine and stool – Note well-being and baby status post feed	
• *Identify clinical clues to poor weight gain:* – *Temperature:* Document temperature, cold peripheries (persistent cold stress), core periphery mismatch (>3°C: Sepsis) – *Jaundice:* High-colored urine, clay stools, jaundice >14 days suggest cholestasis – *Skin:* Cold peripheries, off color, mottling, bleeding from any site, rash, discharge from any site, discoloration suggests bacterial or fungal sepsis – *Infections:* Look for pustules, discharge from any site, feeding, crying during micturition, foul smell discharge, or fever – *Respiratory system:* Breathing difficulty, increased work of breathing, acidotic breathing, color change, audible sounds – *Cardiovascular system*: Color change, breathing difficulty, suck swallow pattern, sweating over forehead, bluish discoloration on crying, upper- and lower-limb peripheral oxygen saturation (SpO_2), femoral pulsations, hyperdynamic precordium, bounding pulses, upper and lower-limb blood pressure (BP), palable liver	

Contd...

Contd...

Step	Tick here
– *Central nervous system:* Activity, sensorium (active, alert, drowsy, irritable, lethargic), cry (shrill, poor, lusty), abnormal movements, or posture – *Gastrointestinal tract:* Vomiting, regurgitation, arching of back, excessive irritability, abdominal distension – *Polyuria*: Urine output >3 mL/kg/h (rental tubular acidosis, diabetes insipidus, Bartter syndrome) – Abnormal odor to body, urine [inborn errors of metabolism (IEM)]	

Note: Some of the important causes of poor weight are:

- *Reduced intake:* Poor lactation, poor suck, neurological abnormal
- *Excess losses:* Vomiting, loose stools, polyuria
- *Increased metabolism:* Infections, systemic diseases

CHAPTER

2.18

Bubble Continuous Positive Airway Pressure Adequacy

Case: Evaluate for bubble continuous positive airway pressure (CPAP) setting adequacy for this 30 weeks, 1.2 kg baby with Respiratory Distress Syndrome (RDS) and on bubble CPAP with pressure of 5 cm, flow of 5 L/min and fraction of inspired oxygen (FiO_2) of 0.30.

OBJECTIVE

At the end of examination for CPAP settings, one should be able to reach following conclusion:

- Note the settings and confirm adequacy

CHECKLIST

Step	*Tick here*
• *Note clinical adequacy:* – Comfortable baby; color pink; regular respiration – No grunt or chest indrawing; breath sounds bilaterally equal – Orogastric tube placed with distal end open	
Note CPAP: • Minimal or no chest recessions, good air entry, bubbles heard in the chest *Note FiO_2:* • Oxygen saturations between 91% and 95% • Color pink *Flow:* • Note the water level in the bubble chamber • Uniform bubbling during breathing *Humidification:* • Servo-controlled humidifier • Temperature displayed is 37°C • Heater wire in the inspiratory limb is present • No condensation in inspiratory limb • Some condensate in the expiratory limb (if not heated wired) *Prongs:* • Snuggly fitting • No erythema or blanching on the alae nasi • There is a gap between the prongs and columella • Prongs fixed to cap and cap is covering the ears • Cap is fixed snuggly to the head	

CHAPTER 2.19

Ventilator Settings

Case: Evaluate for ventilator setting adequacy for this term 3.2 kg infant with meconium aspiration syndrome.

OBJECTIVE

At the end of examination for ventilator setting, one should be able to reach following conclusions:

- Note the ventilator setting and confirm adequacy.
- Note clinical adequacy.

CHECKLIST

Step	*Tick here*
• *Note peak inspiratory pressure (PIP):* Look for chest rise (gentle rise of chest), bilateral equal air entry • *Note positive end-expiratory pressure (PEEP):* Minimal or no chest recessions and chest expansion appropriate (does not look hyperinflated when observed from the side of the baby) • *Notes FiO_2:* Oxygen saturations between 91 and 95% • *Note set rate and patient's rate:* – Each breath of the infant is triggered – Synchrony between ventilator and patient breath • *Note inspiratory time:* – On the flow–time graph, there is some gap between inspiratory and expiratory flow – On the pressure–time graph, the plateau phase is not unusually long • *Flow:* The delivered PIP is as much as the set PIP • *Humidification:* – Servo-controlled humidifier in invasive mode – Temperature displayed is 37°C – Heater wire in the inspiratory limb is present – No condensation in inspiratory limb – Some condensate in the expiratory limb • *Ask for X-ray chest:* – Look for chest expansion with dome of diaphragm between 6 and 8 ribs – Note the position of endotracheal (ET tube) • Check the set ventilator alarm settings • *Notes clinical adequacy:* – Comfortable baby; color pink; regular respiration – No chest indrawing; breath sounds bilaterally equal	

CHAPTER 2.20

Red Reflex Test

Objective: Screening of eye using red reflex test

CHECKLIST

Step	*Tick*
• Introduce self and briefly explain test to parent • Ensure semidarkness, sit at least 1–2 feet away, baby in mother's lap, ensure focus on direct ophthalmoscope is zero • Turn on the direct ophthalmoscope, direct light on each eye and see through the aperture of ophthalmoscope • Inspect each eye separately. Note the presence or absence, symmetry, color, and intensity of reflex • Interpret as normal or abnormal • Counsel and thank parent for need for repeat evaluation • Document the finding	

FREQUENTLY ASKED QUESTIONS

- Is a red, orange, yellow or peach color reflex normal?
  - Yes
- What abnormal reflex would prompt you for referral for ophthalmologic evaluation?
  - Absent reflex, white reflex, or asymmetric reflex
- How to open the baby's eyes?
  - Rock the baby, hold the baby upright
- Till what age is periodic evaluation required?
  - 2 years
- What risk factors should be assessed prior to the test?
  - Prematurity, trisomy 21, family history of strabismus, retinoblastoma, congenital cataracts, or genetic diseases
- What does absent reflex signify?
  - Cataracts, corneal scars, vitreous hemorrhage, or topical eye drops
- What does abnormal size, shape or position of red reflex signify?
  - Aniridia, coloboma of iris, strabismus, dilating drops, trauma

SECTION 3

Clinical Decision Making

CHAPTER

3.1 Jaundice

INTERPRETATION OF FINDINGS

Station 1

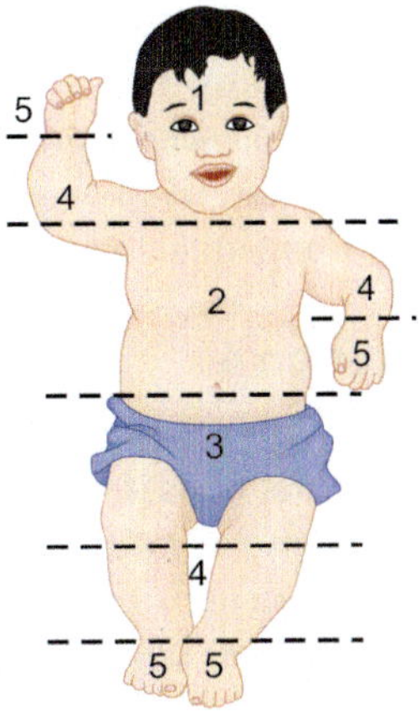

1. **Name two sites for jaundice visualization.**
2. **Identify the staging.**
3. **Name three limitations of this staging.**
4. **Name two postnatal risk factors.**

Ans:

1. Skin, sclera, and mucosa.
2. Kramer's staging.
3. Not applicable for preterm, babies with dark pigmentation, babies exposed to phototherapy (PT) or sunlight, subjective, and do not correlate with severity of jaundice.
4. Breastfeeding inadequacy, sepsis, and polycythemia.

Station 2

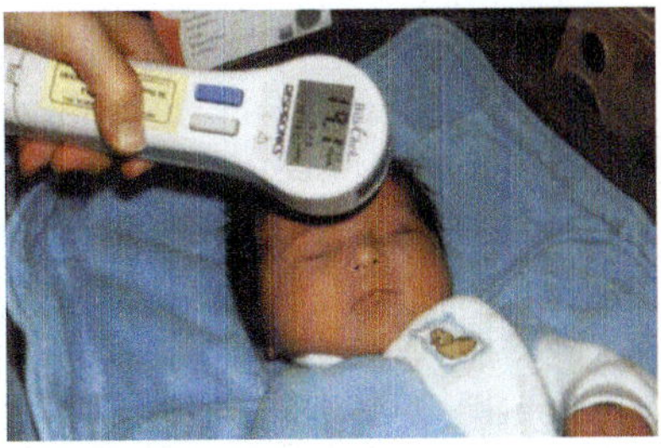

1. **Identify the equipment.**
2. **Name two sites for use.**
3. **Name three limitations of its use.**
4. **What is the cutoff to ask for blood test [total serum bilirubin (TSB)]?**

Ans:

1. Transcutaneous bilirubin meter.
2. Forehead or sternum.
3. Not applicable for babies <35 weeks of gestation, not for babies under PT and not for use in first 24 hours and not for initiating jaundice treatment.
4. TSB >15 mg/dL.

Station 3

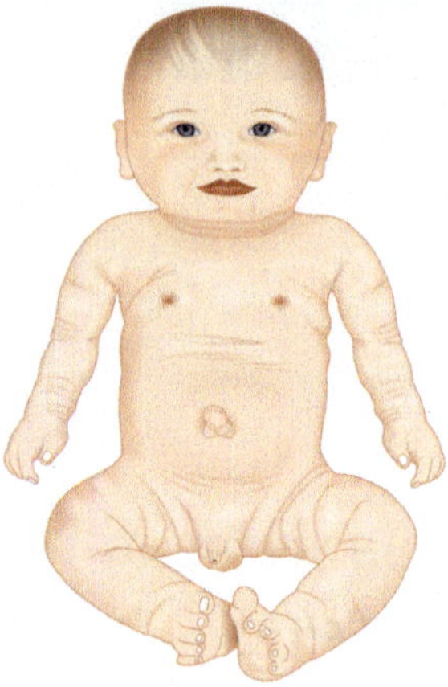

1. **Name five clinical clues to pathological jaundice.**
2. **Name a test to confirm physiologic jaundice.**
3. **Name two conditions which present with mixed hyperbilirubinemia (direct and indirect jaundice).**

Ans:

1. Pallor, plethora, hepatosplenomegaly, high colored urine, clay or pale stools, unstable vital parameters, evidence of sepsis, e.g., thermal instability, poor suck, feeding difficulty, rash, foul odor, bleeding tendency, altered sensorium, and abnormal cry.
2. No test. It is a diagnosis of exclusion.
3. Congenital hypothyroidism, sepsis, and galactosemia.

Station 4

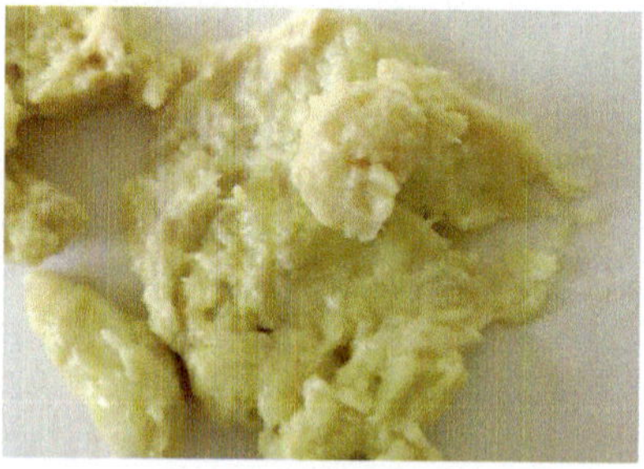

1. **What is the diagnosis?**
2. **What does it indicate?**
3. **Name a gold standard test to confirm?**
4. **Within what period of time should you intervene surgically?**

Ans:

1. Clay stool or pale stools.
2. Indicates intrahepatic or extrahepatic biliary tract obstruction.
3. Liver biopsy (direct bilirubin >1 mg/dL, urinary bile salts, and bile pigments positive).
4. As early as possible but within 60 days.

Station 5

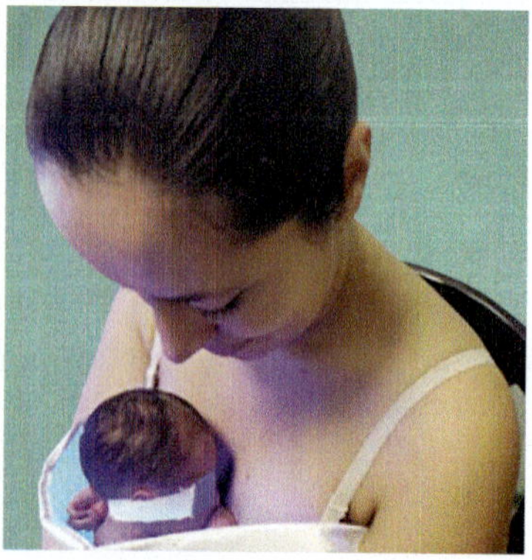

1. **Identify the type of PT.**
2. **Name two benefits of this PT.**
3. **Name two drawbacks of this PT.**
4. **Name four systemic factors compromising blood brain barrier.**

Ans:

1. Fiber-optic PT.

2. *Benefits:* No separation between mother and baby, kangaroo mother care (KMC), breastfeeding promoting, and thermal support.
3. *Drawbacks:* Not for intensive PT, not for large babies, and costly.
4. Hypoxia, hypercarbia, hypoglycemia, systemic sepsis, meningitis, thermal instability, acidosis, and hypoalbuminemia.

Station 6

1. **Identify the chart.**
2. **Name two treatable causes of cholestasis.**
3. **Name gold standard for diagnosis of biliary atresia.**

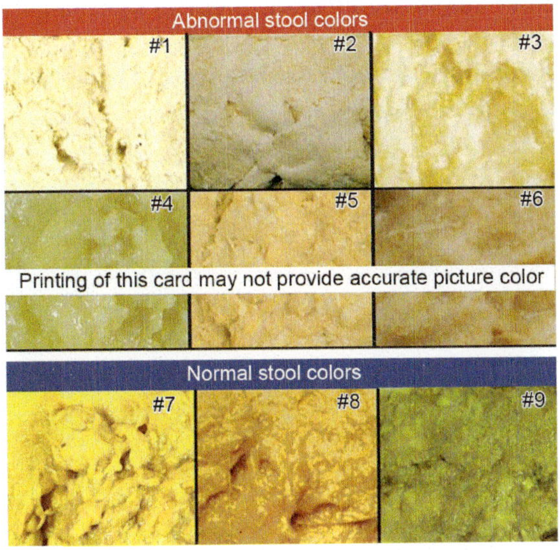

Ans:

1. Stool color chart for screening of conjugated jaundice.
2. Galactosemia and congenital hypothyroidism.
3. Intraoperative cholangiogram.

Station 7

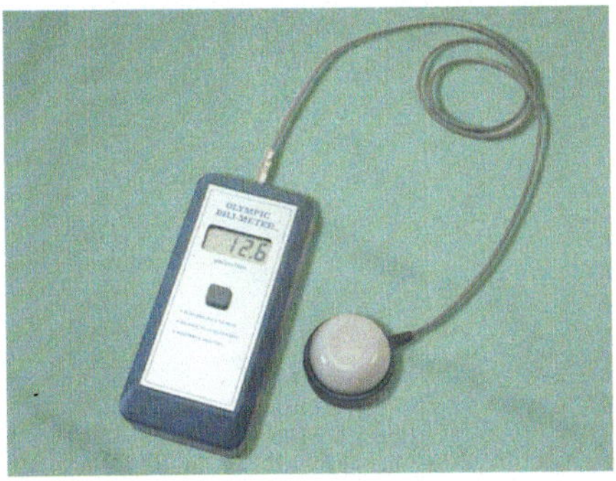

1. **Identify the equipment.**
2. **Name four factors affecting PT efficacy.**
3. **Give two examples of conventional PT.**
4. **Name four neurotoxic risk factors for jaundice.**

Ans:

1. Bilimeter.

2. Type (spectrum) of light, irradiance, area of exposure, and hydration of the baby.
3. Blue-white PT, compact fluorescent lamp (CFL), light emitting diode (LED), and fiber-optic PT.
4. Sepsis, hemolytic jaundice, hypoalbuminemia, and clinical instability in the last 24 hours.

Station 8

1. **Name four neurotoxic risk factors for jaundice.**
2. **Name four predischarge risk factors for significant jaundice.**
3. **Name components of bilirubin-induced neurological dysfunction (BIND) score.**
4. **What bilirubin rise should raise suspicion of hemolysis?**

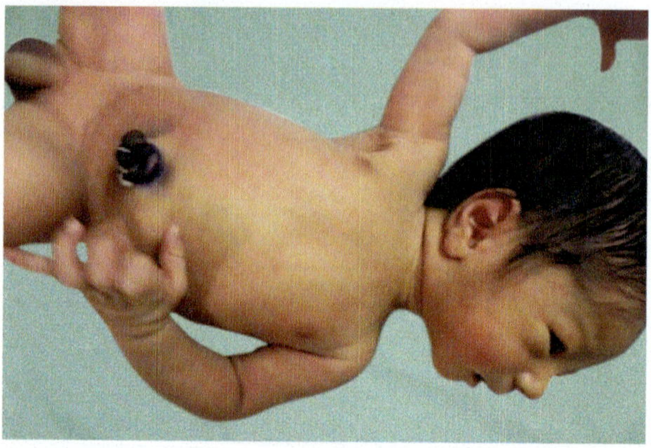

Ans:

1. Albumin <3g/dL, sepsis, unstable over last 24 hours, and hemolysis.
2. Preterm, suboptimal breastfeeding, infant of diabetic mother, trisomy 21, onset of jaundice within 24 hours, and previous sibling requiring jaundice therapy.
3. Mental status, muscle tone, and cry.
4. >0.3 mg/dL/hour in first 24 hours and >0.2 mg/dL/hour after 24 hours.

3.2

CHAPTER

Cholestasis

INTERPRETATION OF FINDINGS

Diagnosis of Cholestasis

1. Name any two clinical clues to neonatal cholestasis.
2. What value of conjugate bilirubin should raise suspicion of cholestasis?
3. Name any two features of liver cell failure.
4. Name any three etiologies that present as liver cell failure in a newborn.
5. What is the age at which evaluation of cholestasis is mandated in a jaundiced newborn and what is the age before which definitive management of biliary atresia is recommended?

Answers:

1. Jaundice lasting for >2 weeks, yellow sclera, urine staining diapers, and pale stools
2. Conjugate bilirubin >1 mg/dL.
3. Coagulopathy not corrected with vitamin K, encephalopathy, and/or ascites.
4. Infections [bacterial, cytomegalovirus (CMV), and herpes], tyrosinemia, galactosemia, gestational alloimmune liver disease, bile acid synthetic defects, and mitochondrial disorders.
5. 2 weeks and 60 days.

Clinical Evaluation

1. Name three classical clinical features of infant with biliary atresia.
2. Name two cholestasis liver diseases associated with syndromic features.
3. What is the likely etiology in a newborn presenting with liver cell failure, moderate hepatomegaly, transaminases elevated [52 IU/mL and 76 IU/mL of aspartate transaminase (AST) and alanine transaminase (ALT)], ferritin 1,450 ng/mL, elevated alpha fetoprotein, and low fibrinogen?

Answers:

1. Well looking and thriving child, firm liver, pale stools, and urine staining the diaper.
2. Alagille syndrome, Zellweger syndrome, and Smith-Lemli-Opitz syndrome.
3. Gestational alloimmune liver disease.

Match the Clinical Finding (One or More) with the Etiology

i. Hypothyroidism	a. Cataract
ii. Hypopituitarism	b. *Escherichia coli* sepsis
iii. Progressive familial intrahepatic cholestasis (PFIC)	c. Hypoglycemia on feeding
iv. Bile acid synthetic defects	d. Midline defects
v. Gestational alloimmune liver disease (GALD)	e. Butterfly vertebrae
vi. Alagille syndrome	f. Wide posterior fontanelle
vii. Galactosemia	g. Pruritus
	h. Early, low or normal gamma-glutamyl transferase (GGT)
	i. Neonatal liver failure

Answers:

i.–f, ii.–d, iii.–g and h, iv.–g and h, v–i, vi–e, vii–a and b

Investigations

1. Name a test to identify acuity of liver disease.
2. Name a test to identify obstructive liver disease.
3. Name a test to identify chronicity of liver disease.
4. Name a test to prognosticate liver disease.
5. What is the classical sign in ultrasound of biliary atresia?
6. What are the diseases that may mimic biliary atresia on the liver biopsy?
7. What is the gold standard for diagnosis of biliary atresia?
8. Name a condition diagnosed by matrix metalloproteinase 7 levels and transient elastography.

Answers:

1. AST and ALT.
2. Alkaline phosphatase and GGT.
3. Serum albumin.
4. Prothrombin time.
5. Triangular cord sign.
6. PFIC, sclerosing cholangitis, cystic fibrosis, and Alagille syndrome.
7. Liver biopsy.
8. Biliary atresia.

Management

1. What is the procedure of choice for surgical management of extrahepatic biliary atresia (EHBA)?
2. What is the treatment of choice for PFIC?
3. Match the treatment with the etiology of cholestasis:

i. Nitisinone	a. Bile acid synthetic defect
ii. Intravenous immunoglobulin (IVIG)	b. Tyrosinemia
iii. Sugar-free diet	c. GALD
iv. Oral cholic acid	d. Fructosemia

4. Write the doses of following for cholestasis in newborn:
   i. Vitamin A, D, E, and K
   ii. Water-soluble vitamins

Answers:

1. Portoenterostomy or Kasai surgery.
2. Ursodeoxycholic acid (UDCA), biliary diversion, and liver transplantation.
3. i. *Nitisinone:* Tyrosinemia
   ii. *IVIG:* GALD
   iii. *Sugar-free diet:* Fructosemia
   iv. *Oral cholic acid:* Bile acid synthetic defects
4. i. *Vitamin A:* 5,000–25,000 IU/d, Vitamin D: 400–1,200 IU/day, Vitamin E: 50–400 IU/day or 15–25 IU/kg/day, Vitamin K: 2–5 mg IM, SC, or IV 4 weekly.
   ii. *Water-soluble vitamins:* One to two times the recommended dietary allowance (RDA).

CHAPTER

3.3 Seizures

INTERPRETATION OF FINDINGS

Seizure Identification

1. **What is the gold standard for diagnosis of neonatal seizure as per the International League Against Epilepsy (ILAE)?**
2. **Name three clinical clues to differentiate seizure from jitteriness.**
3. **Name two categories of neonatal seizures as per ILAE.**
4. **Name two seizures with good electroencephalogram (EEG) correlation.**
5. **Name two seizures with poor EEG correlation.**
6. **How to assess seizure burden as per the ILAE.**
7. **Name two metabolic causes of in utero seizures.**

Ans:

1. EEG.
2. Seizures are stimulus insensitive, associated with abnormal eye and facial movements, and vitals sign changes.
3. EEG only and electroclinical seizures. Electroclinical further classified as motor (automatisms, clonic, epileptic spasms, myoclonic, and tonic), nonmotor (autonomic and behavior arrest), sequential, and unclassified.
4. Seizures with EEG correlate are focal clonic and focal tonic.
5. Seizures with poor EEG correlation are automatisms and generalized tonic seizures.
6. Seizure burden is assessed from the duration of seizure activity on the EEG from the total hours of recording.
7. Pyridoxine dependent seizures and nonketotic hyperglycinemia.

Amplitude-integrated Electroencephalography

1. **What is the diagnosis on this amplitude integrated electroencephalography (aEEG)?**
2. **Name two reassuring pattern (normal brain) on aEEG.**
3. **Which seizures are not identified on aEEG?**
4. **Name three prognostic patterns on aEEG.**

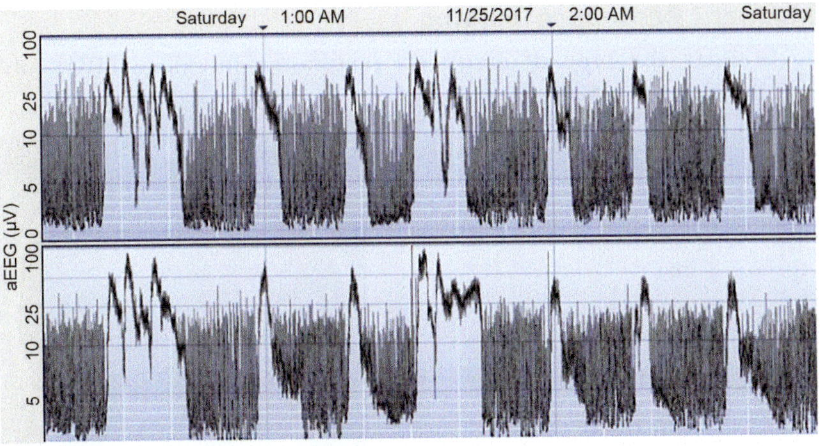

Ans:

1. Sudden rise in low amplitude accompanied by sudden rise in high amplitude.
2. Amplitude between 10 and 25 microV and presence of sleep wave cycle pattern.
3. Brief seizures and automatisms.
4. Background activity predicts prognosis: Low voltage (lower <5 and upper <10), loss of sleep wave cycle, and discontinuous waveform.

Clinical Clues to Seizures

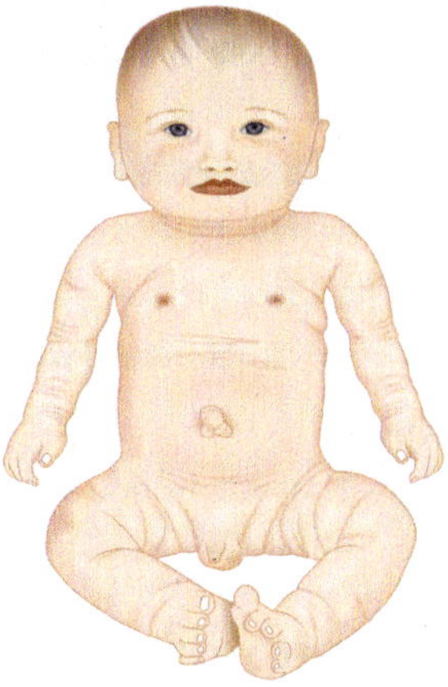

1. **What is the clinical clue to channelopathies?**
2. **What are the clinical clues to pyridoxine dependent seizures?**
3. **Match the etiology [hypoxic ischemic encephalopathy (HIE), inborn error of metabolism (IEM), hypoglycemia, and meningitis) to the clinical condition:**
   a. **Infant of diabetic mother (IDM)**
   b. **Abnormal nonstress test (NST)**
   c. **Vomiting, acidosis, and encephalopathy**
   d. **Maternal premature rupture of membrane (PROM)**

Ans:

1. Unprovoked seizures presenting with sequential seizures (progression of clonic to tonic to myoclonic seizure).
2. Myoclonic or spasms, grimacing, and burst suppression on the EEG.
3. A—hypoglycemia, b—HIE, c—IEM, and d—meningitis

Magnetic Resonance Imaging

1. **Identify the type of magnetic resonance imaging (MRI) and characteristic pattern?**

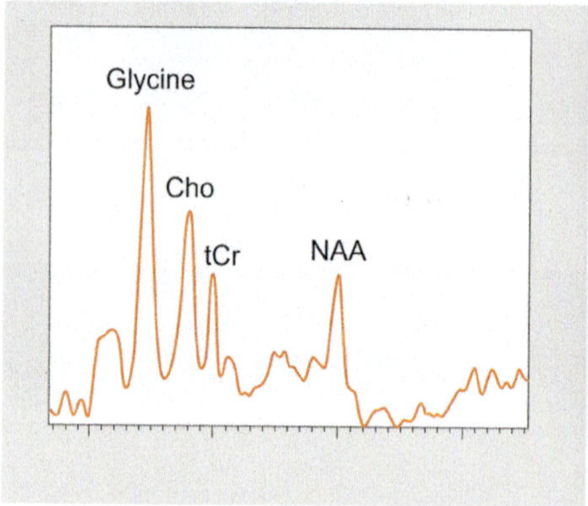

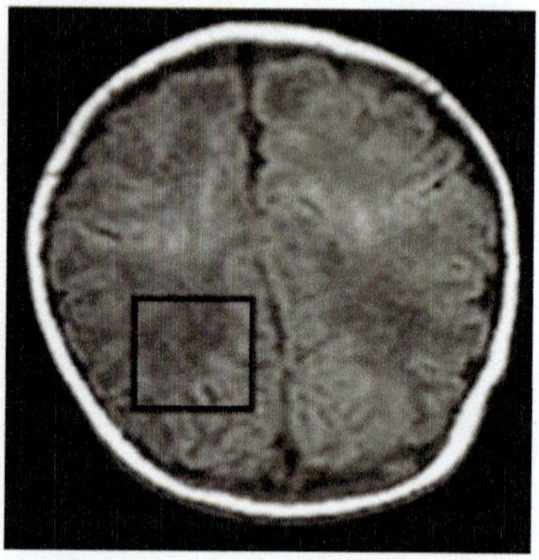

2. **Name three metabolic disorders with these MRI findings.**
3. **Match the MRI with the etiology of seizure. (HIE, hypoglycemia, and viral infections)**

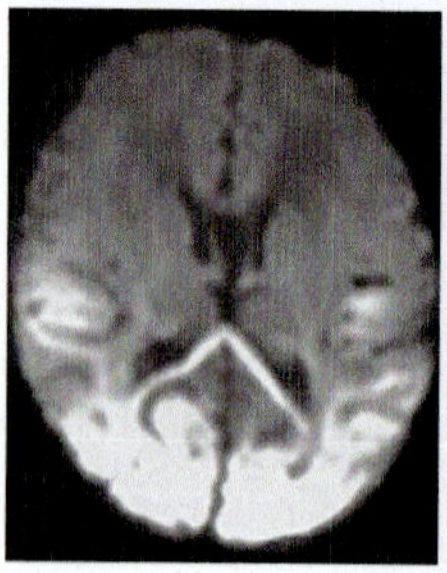

Fig. 1

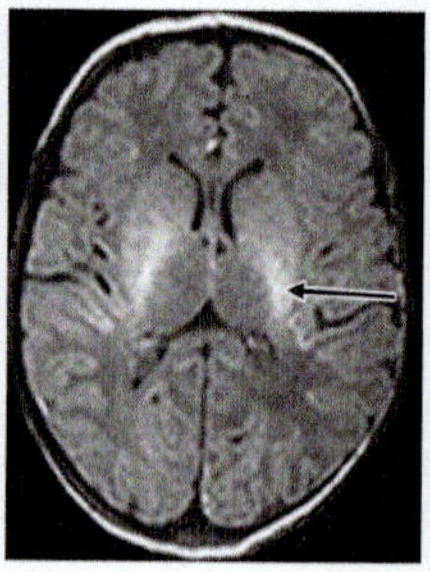

Fig. 2

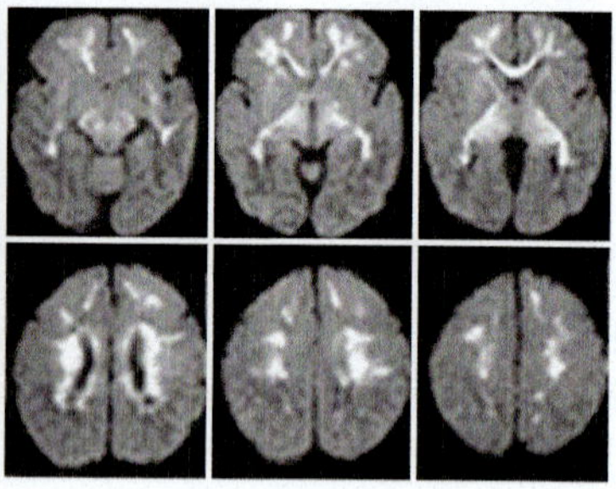

Fig. 3

4. **What MRI sequence/type is required for a term infant with severe dehydration and multiple seizures?**

Ans:

1. MR spectroscopy showing elevated glycine peak.
2. Nonketotic hyperglycinemia, mitochondrial disorders, and creatine deficiency.
3. Hypoglycemia **(Fig. 1)**, HIE **(Fig. 2)**, and Viral infections (entero- or parechovirus) **(Fig. 3)**.
4. MRI venography for identifying cerebral venous thrombosis.

Management

1. **Management of neonatal seizures as per the ILAE:**
   a. **What is the first-line antiepileptic drug (AED) for treatment?**
   b. **Name any three drugs used for second-line AEDs.**
   c. **What AEDs are preferred in a newborn suspected with channelopathies and in which condition these AEDs should not be given?**
   d. **The decision to discontinue AED in acute asymptomatic seizures without evidence of neonatal onset epilepsy is based on: (i) EEG, (ii) MRI, (iii) Neurologic examination, (iv) None of the above**
   e. **What is the second-line AED in a newborn with congenital heart disease?**

Ans:

a. Phenobarbitone.
b. Fosphenytoin/phenytoin, leviracetam, lidocaine, and midazolam.
c. Phenytoin/leviracetam and Dravet syndrome.
d. iv. Following cessation of acute symptomatic seizures (electroclinical or electrographic) without evidence for neonatal onset epilepsy, antiseizure medications should be discontinued before discharge home, regardless of MRI or EEG findings.
e. Leviracetam.

CHAPTER 3.4

Sepsis

INTERPRETATION OF FINDINGS

Clinical Features of Sepsis

1. **Name any five clinical predictor signs of severe neonatal sepsis as per Young Infant Study Group.**
2. **Match the clinical scenario.**

a. Early-onset sepsis	1. Symptomatic with isolation of organism from sterile site
b. Suspected sepsis	2. Clinical manifestations within 72 hours of birth
c. Clinical sepsis	3. Clinical and laboratory findings of sepsis present, but failure to isolate the causative microorganism
d. Proven sepsis	4. Presence of risk factors in an asymptomatic newborn
	5. Symptomatic and laboratory findings absent

3. **Name two independent markers for late onset sepsis.**

Ans.

1. Predictive signs of severe sepsis in the first 2 months of life are history of difficulty feeding, history of convulsions, movement only when stimulated, respiratory rate ≥60 breaths per minute, severe chest indrawing, axillary temperature ≥37.5°C, axillary temperature <35.5°C.
2. a-2, b-4, c-3, d-1
3. Independent markers for late-onset sepsis are appearance of thrombocytopenia and poor perfusion.

Regarding Neonatal Herpes Simplex Infection

1. Name the typical histologic features on Tzanck smear.
2. What is the duration of intravenous acyclovir therapy for skin-eye-mouth (SEM) disease and encephalitis?
3. Name two tests that should be done in all confirmed infants irrespective of disease severity.

Ans.

1. Multinucleated giant cells and eosinophilic intranuclear inclusions.
2. 14 days and 21 days.
3. Neuroimaging and ophthalmic evaluation.

Investigations

1. **Calculate the immature to the total neutrophil ratio (I:T) ratio if complete blood count (CBC) shows white blood cell (WBC) 18,000/mm^3, N45, myelocytes 2%, metamyelocytes 3%, band forms 5%, and platelets are 1.8 lakhs/mm^3.**
2. **Identify the cells on the blood picture.**

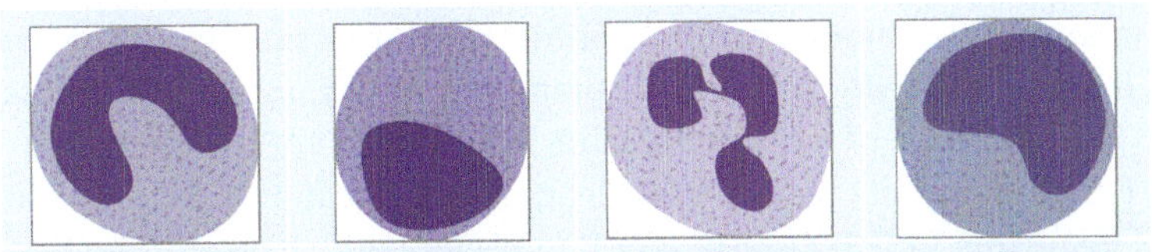

A B C D

3. **What are the cerebrospinal fluid (CSF) features suggestive of meningitis?**
4. **If the positive likelihood ratio and negative likelihood ratio is 3.5 and 0.5 for C-reactive protein (CRP), what is the post-test probability in a newborn with cold peripheries, dusky peripheries, poor feeding, and abdominal distension where the pretest probability of infection is 20%?**
5. **Differentiating features between CRP and procalcitonin in the diagnosis of neonatal sepsis.**

Ans.

1. IT ratio is 2 + 3 + 5/45 + 2 + 3 + 5 = 10/55 = 0.18.
2. (A) Band form, (B) myelocyte, (C) mature neutrophil, (D) metamyelocyte.
3. CSF protein >150 mg/dL in preterm and >100 mg/dL in term infant and cell count >15/mm^3 with predominant neutrophils.
4. The calculation involves:
   - Pretest probability is 0.20
   - Pretest odds is 1/5
   - Post odds if CRP positive is 1/5*3.5, i.e., 3.5/5 and post-test odds if CRP negative is 1/5*0.5 which is 1/10
   - Post-test probability if CRP positive is 3.5/8.5 (41%) and if CRP negative the probability is 1/11 which is 9%
5. CRP versus procalcitonin:
   - CRP raises later than procalcitonin
   - Procalcitonin is more specific for bacterial infections
   - Procalcitonin is a predictor of severity of infection
   - Procalcitonin is better marker for antibiotic duration

Blood Cultures

1. **Name four strategies to improve the yield of blood culture.**
2. **Name four causes of false-negative blood culture.**
3. **Name any two features of culture contamination. What is the expected contamination rate among neonatal blood cultures?**

Ans.

1. Strategies for improving yield of blood culture—1 mL of blood, obtain culture before starting of antibiotics, new venipuncture, first sample from hub of needle, avoid indwelling catheters, hand hygiene, automated culture techniques (Bactec and BacT Alert), ratio of blood to culture medium should be >1:10.
2. Blood culture may be sterile despite infection if insufficient sample, maternal antibiotic therapy, antibiotic prior to sampling, low bacteria load, slow growing bacteria, laboratory error, or nonbacterial illness.
3. The features of contamination are identification of a skin flora (staphylococcal epidermidis), delayed identification (>5 days), different organisms in two culture medium if two culture taken. The expected contamination should be <3% among all cultures obtained.

Match the Interpretation of a Blood Culture Report

a. Susceptible (S)	i. There is a high likelihood of therapeutic failure even when there is increased exposure.
b. Susceptible (I)	ii. There is a high likelihood of therapeutic success using a standard dosing regimen of the agent.
c. Resistant (R)	iii. There is a high likelihood of therapeutic success because exposure to the agent is increased by adjusting the dosing regimen or by its concentration at the site of infection.
d. Efficiency ratio	iv. Approximate drug concentration that can be reasonably achieved safely in the plasma using the normal dose and route of administration of the drug.
	v. Minimum concentration of the drug that will inhibit the in vitro growth of the organism and is specific to the organism isolated and the drug.
	vi. It is ratio of breakpoint MIC/MIC.

Ans. a-ii, b-iii, c-i, d-vi

Antibiotics

1. Name any two factors that influence the choice of empiric antibiotic for suspected early-onset sepsis (EOS)/late-onset sepsis (LOS).
2. Name any two mechanisms of antimicrobial drug resistance.
3. Match the drug resistance among microbes.

a. Multidrug-resistant (MDR)	i. Nonsusceptibility to at least one antibiotic within three or more antibiotic categories
b. Extensively drug-resistant (XDR)	ii. Nonsusceptibility to all antibiotics in all categories
c. Pandrug-resistant (PanDR)	iii. Nonsusceptibility to at least one antibiotic in all categories but only for two or fewer antibiotic categories

Ans.

1. *The site of infection:* Choose the drug that is likely to concentrate the tissue of infection. Expected Organism: Choose a drug that cover gram-positive infections if the infant has a boil, a pustule or omphalitis. Choose a drug for which most previous microbes were susceptible (60–80%).
2. The mechanisms by which a microbe develops resistance are efflux pumps, antibiotic inactivation (penicillin and cephalosporin), change in target site (trimethoprim-sulfisoxazole), modification of metabolic pathways to circumvent antibiotic effect, overproduction of antibiotic target site, and biofilm formation.
3. a-i, b-iii, c-ii

MRI/CT Diagnosis

Match the neuroimaging with the organism:

Case A

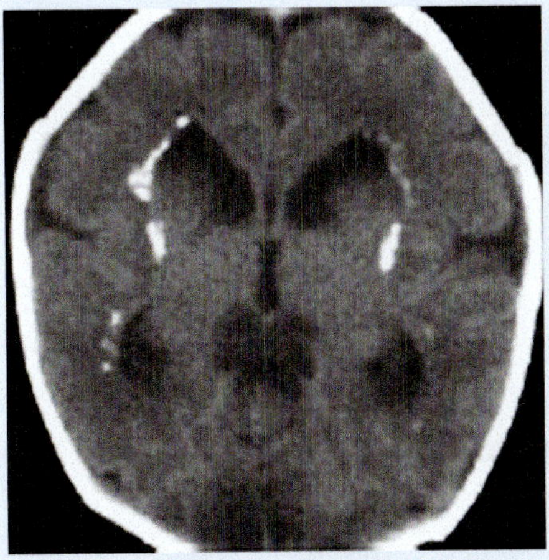

Case B

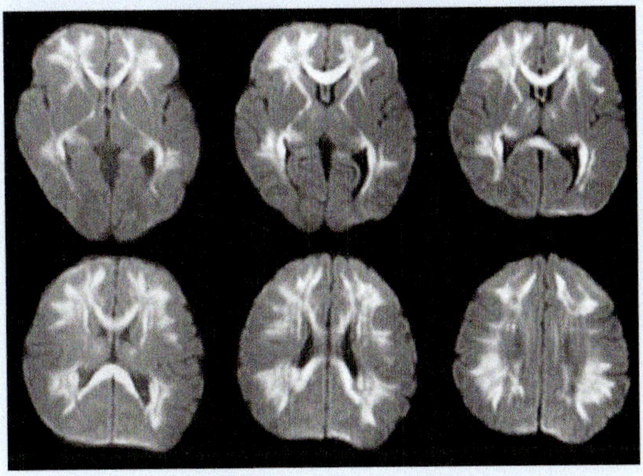

a. Congenital toxoplasmosis
b. Congenital human immunodeficiency virus (HIV)
c. Congenital cytomegalovirus (CMV)
d. Enterovirus or parechovirus infections
e. Herpes infection
f. Abscesses (Citrobacter)
g. *Candida albicans*
h. Parvovirus

Contd...

Contd...

Case C

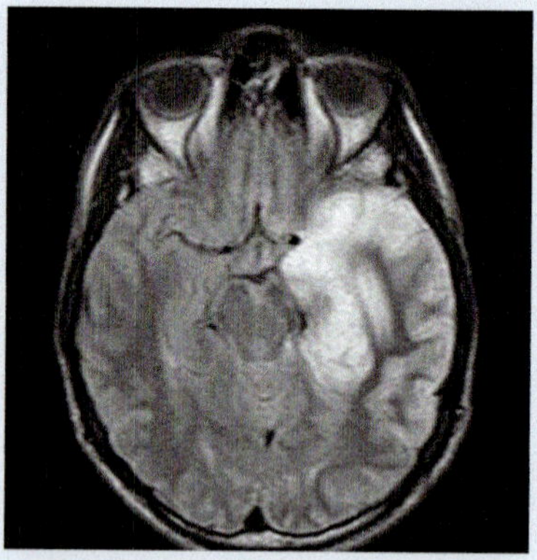

Case D

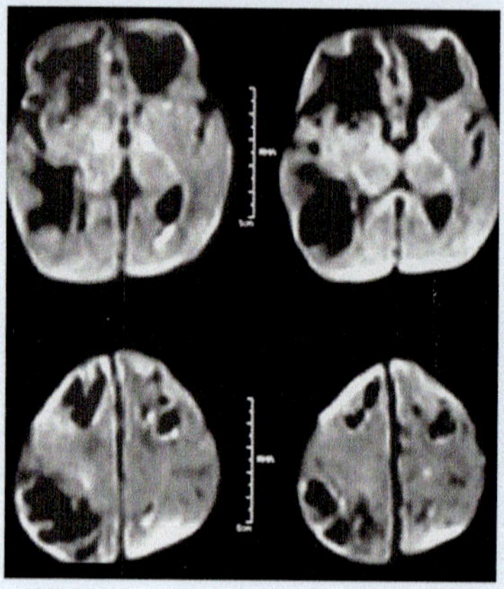

Ans. A-c, B-d, C-e, D-f

CHAPTER

3.5

Surgery

SPOTS

1.

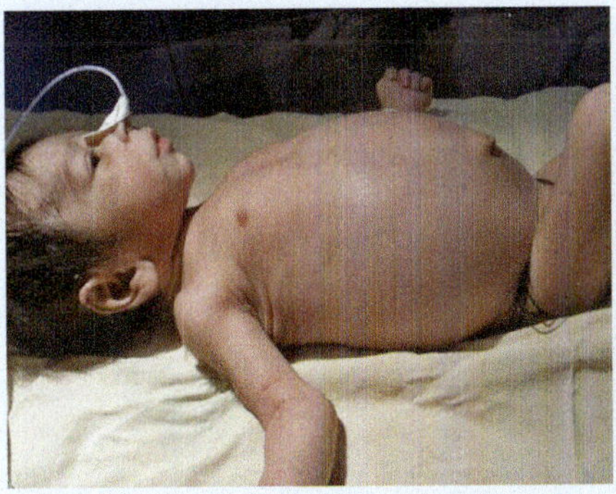

a. Name two nonsurgical causes of distended abdomen.
b. Name a surgical emergency without abdominal distention or bilious vomiting.
c. By what postnatal age does air reach the all of the small bowel and rectum?
d. How is dilated bowel loop defined?
e. How do you differentiate high versus low gut obstruction on X-ray?
f. Name a definitive test to differentiate small from large bowel.
g. Name two pathological conditions with absent rectal air.
h. Name two findings of perforation in utero.
i. By what gestation does bowel return back to the abdominal cavity?
j. Name the most frequent cause of upper gut obstruction.
k. Name the definitive test for Hirschsprung's disease.
l. Presence of bowel anomaly should prompt a systemic search for which conditions?

Ans.

a. Hepatosplenomegaly, ascites, gaseous distention, and neoplasm.
b. Malrotation of gut, esophageal atresia, duodenal atresia, and jejunal atresia.

c. 12 hours and 24 hours.
d. Bowel measures more than the interpedicular width of L2.
e. Up to three dilated small bowel loops indicates high obstruction, more than three dilated loops indicates low obstruction.
f. Lower gastrointestinal (GI) contrast.
g. Meconium ileus and Hirschsprung's disease.
h. Ascites, free air, and abdominal wall calcification.
i. 10th week.
j. Jejunal atresia.
k. Bowel biopsy.
l. VACTERL search.

2.

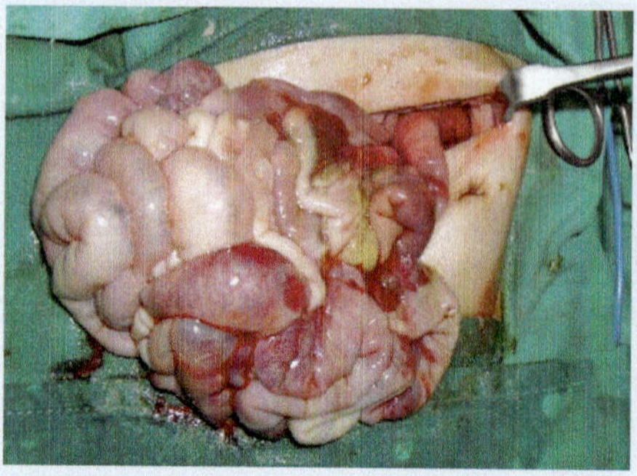

a. Identify the pathology in this preterm.
b. What best surgical intervention can be done at this stage?
c. What postoperative nutritional support would you advise?
d. Name two complications of surgery.
e. What long-term gut problem do you anticipate?

Ans.

a. Extensive areas of ischemia, necrosis, and gangrene of small intestine.
b. Ileostomy.
c. Total parenteral nutrition.
d. Stricture, abscess, short bowel syndrome, and recurrence of necrotizing enterocolitis (NEC).
e. Short bowel syndrome.

3.

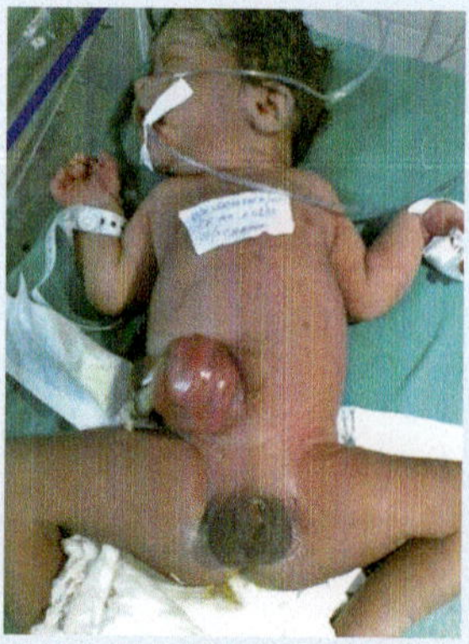

a. What is the diagnosis?
b. How do you grade severity?
c. Name the most common syndrome associated with it.
d. What is the prognosis in this infant with no associated anomaly?

Ans.

a. Omphalocele—mass at the site of the umbilical cord insertion and covered by a membrane.
b. Defect in the abdominal wall >5 cm is major or giant omphalocele
c. Beckwith-Wiedemann syndrome.
d. With small defects, survival rate is >80%. Presence of liver, giant defects, or associated genetic conditions have guarded prognosis.

4.

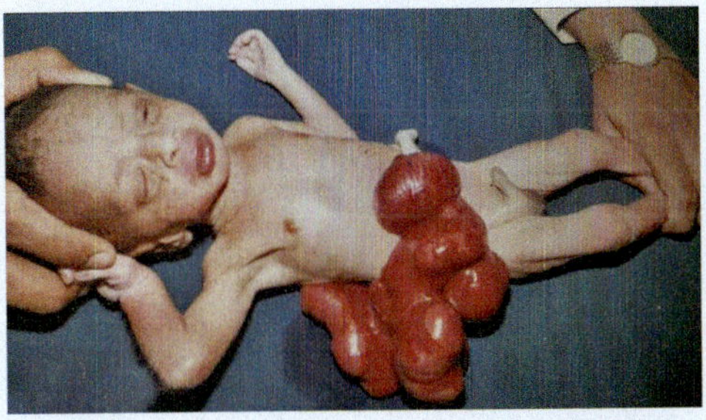

a. What is the diagnosis?
b. Name a clue on maternal blood screening during pregnancy.
c. What is the most common associated ultrasound finding?
d. How do you stratify the condition at birth?
e. Name four interventions to stabilize at birth.

Ans.

a. Gastroschisis—paraumbilical abdominal wall defect with protrusion of the bowel through the defect without a covering membrane.
b. Elevated serum alpha fetoprotein.
c. Intrauterine growth restriction (IUGR) (60%). Associated malformations or genetic causes are rare.
d. Simple (75%) or complex (25%) based on presence or absence of gut pathology, viz., intestinal atresia, stenosis, bowel perforation, necrosis, malrotation, or volvulus.
e. Thermal care, cover defect with sterile cloth and place in a sterile bag such as used blood bag, place orogastric tube, and intravenous (IV) fluid.

5. Match the column with abdominal X-ray changes and clinical condition.

a. No distal bowel gas	i. Polyhydramnios
b. Curled up feeding tube with gasless abdomen	ii. Malrotation
c. Double bubble sign	iii. Esophageal atresia with no tracheoesophageal fistula
d. Dilated stomach with distal bowel gas present	iv. Esophageal atresia with distal tracheoesophageal fistula
e. Corkscrew or reversed 3 sign	v. Duodenal web
f. Triple bubble shadow	vi. Complete obstruction
g. Soap bubble appearance	vii. Malrotation with volvulus
	viii. Jejunal atresia
	ix. Meconium ileus
	x. Hirschsprung's disease

Ans. a-vi, b-iii, c-i, d-v, e-vii, f-viii, g-ix

CHAPTER

3.6

Clinical Spots

SPOTS

1.

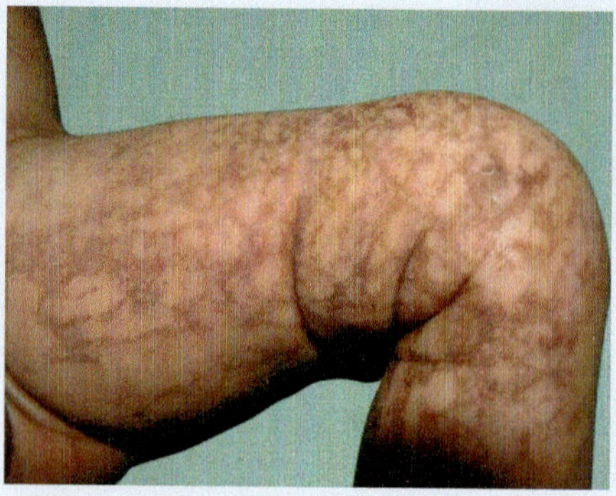

a. Identify the skin lesion.
b. Name two risk outcomes in first year of life.
c. What is the mode of inheritance?
d. What does eye involvement indicate?
e. Name the four stages of skin involvement.

Ans.

a. Incontinentia pigmenti—swirl-like hyperpigmented lesions following the lines of Blaschko.
b. Stroke, seizures, vision loss, and developmental delay.
c. X-linked dominant.
d. Associated neurologic disorder.
e. Atrophic, hyperpigmented, vesicular, and verrucous

2.

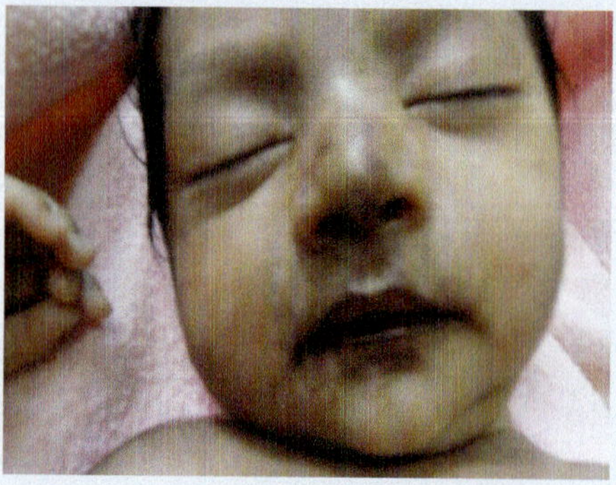

a. Identify the infection causing typical skin lesion.
b. Why do these babies have paradoxical cry—cries on handling and remain quiet when alone?
c. How do you confirm the diagnosis?
d. How does it differ from dengue infection clinically?

Ans.

a. Chikungunya—classical perioral hyperpigmentation.
b. Due to severe bone and muscle inflammation.
c. Polymerase chain reaction (PCR) or immunoglobulin G/immunoglobulin M (IgG/IgM) anti-chikungunya virus (CHIKV)
d. Infrequent hemorrhagic manifestations, no shock, no evidence of gallbladder hydrops or effusions.

3.

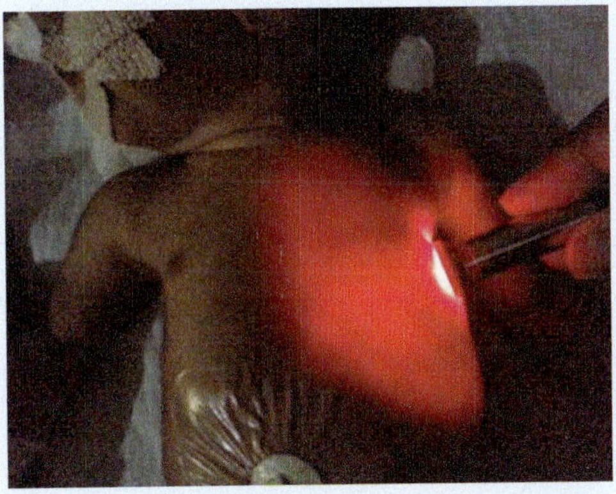

a. Identify the emergency procedure shown.
b. Name four nonemergency indications.
c. Name two conditions with false-negative results.
d. Name two conditions with false-positive results.
e. Name four brain disorders that can be detected.

Ans.

a. Transillumination test for chest.
b. Localize artery or vein for cannulation, aspiration of bladder, skull transillumination for screening of macrocephaly, differentiate cystic from solid mass, serial follow-up of air leak, and abdominal distention evaluation (ascites, pneumoperitoneum, cyst, cystic kidney, and hydronephrosis).
c. Subcutaneous fat and edema.
d. Congenital lobar emphysema and pneumomediastinum.
e. Subdural effusion, subdural hematoma, hydrocephalus, hydranencephaly, and porencephaly.

SECTION 4

Interpretation of Findings

CHAPTER 4.1

TABCD Approach Template

Case: B/o Asha, ___________ weight and gestation, ___________ delivery to primi is brought from ___________ with ________________. How do you approach and stabilize this newborn?

Task:
- Examine the patient with temperature, airway, breathing, circulation, coma, convulsion and dehydration (TABCD) approach
- Identify the problem and give differential diagnosis
- Lay down priorities in management
- You are *not* required to take history of the patient

Duration: 10 minutes

Step	***Tick here***
Basics: • Wash hands, ensure asepsis as required • Introduce self and role • Confirm patient identity • Explain you are here to examine • Gain consent from care giver	
Are there any *"life-threatening"* signs *Ask:* Is there any apnea, gasping, cyanosis, seizure, or nonresponsiveness *Rationale:* If any present, suggest life-threatening emergency *Action:* Skip assessment, call for help, and proceed to resuscitation	
Thermal assessment: *Ask:* Check for temperature *Rationale:* Hypothermia may cause hypoglycemia, hypoxia, and acidosis. Thermal instability may suggest sepsis. *Interpret:* Hypothermia (<36.5°C) and hyperthermia (>37.5°C) *Action:* Ensures baby is kept under warmer with skin probe set at 36.5°C.	
Airway assessment: *Ask:* • Is there spontaneous breathing and visible secretions • Any audible sounds	

Contd...

Contd...

Step	*Tick here*
Rationale: If breathing spontaneously, no secretions or audible sound, suggest patent airway. Visible secretions or stridor suggest partial airway block. Apnea suggests blocked airway. *Interpret:* Patent airway, partial block, or complete airway block. *Action:* Ensure "sniffing position". Do a quick suction if partial block and reposition the airway. Consider intubation if no spontaneous breathing.	
Breathing assessment: *Ask:* • Notes respiratory rate, chest retractions, air entry, breath sounds • Notes the mental status • Documents pulse oximeter *Rationale:* Identify tachypnea (>60/min), bradypnea (<30/min), gasping (poor respiratory efforts), impending respiratory failure (increased work of breathing with altered sensorium) identify respiratory distress as mild (subcostal indrawing), moderate (intercostal indrawing) or severe (suprasternal–supraclavicular indrawing, and grunt), identify mental status as alert, drowsy but arousable, nonresponsive, identify hypoxia [oxygen saturation (SpO_2) <90%) in room air *Interpret:* Normal, respiratory distress, and respiratory failure *Action:* Monitor with pulse oximetry. Ensure temperature is 36.5°C. Does a quick oral suction. Keeps baby in "sniffing position". Asks to reassess every few minutes. Stabilizes on oxygen using nasal prongs at 2 L/min to target oxygen saturation of 91–95%. Considers noninvasive support if hypoxia still persists. Considers intubation if no spontaneous breathing or recurrent apnea or gasping.	
Circulatory assessment: *Ask:* • Notes on heart rate (HR), peripheral pulses, color, capillary refill time (CRT), and skin temperature • Notes on the mental status • Notes on blood pressure (BP) and urine output *Rationale:* Bradycardia (HR <100 beats/min), tachycardia (HR >160 beats/min), pulses weak, bounding or normal, color–pale, dusky, or pink, CRT >3 seconds as prolonged, cold skin is abnormal, note mental status as alert, drowsy but arousable, nonresponsive, systolic BP less than the mean gestational age is hypotension, urine output as oliguria if (<1 cc/kg/hour) *Interpret:* Normal, compensated shock (poor perfusion with normal BP), and hypotensive shock (poor perfusion with low BP) *Action:* Fluid bolus, inotropes, monitor BP, and consider point-of-care ultrasound (POCUS)	

Contd...

Contd...

Step	***Tick here***
Dextrose assessment: *Ask:* Check for Glucostix *Rationale:* The threshold for treating hypoglycemia in the first 4 hours is venous blood glucose values of <25 mg%, between 4 and 24 hours <35 mg% and beyond 24 hours is <45 mg%. *Interpret:* Normo- or hypoglycemia. *Action:* Identifies if baby is symptomatic or asymptomatic. For asymptomatic baby offers supervised feeding and for symptomatic baby offers glucose push and continuous glucose infusion rate of 6–8 mg/kg/min	
Problem identification: • Hypothermia or hyperthermia • Blocked or partially blocked airway • Hypoxia or hyperoxia • Respiratory distress (mild, moderate, or severe) or respiratory failure • Shock (compensated or hypotensive) • Drowsy but arousable and nonresponsive	
Plan of action: • Hospitalize and stabilize under warmer • Place baby on a multichannel monitor • Secure intravenous (IV) line. Collect blood for glucose and culture to rule out sepsis • Start maintenance fluid drip • Monitor sensorium, respiratory, and circulatory status periodically • Reassess by next 30 minutes • Counsel parents and take details of history	

CHAPTER

4.1A

Respiratory Distress

Case: B/o Asha, 34 weeks, 1.8 kg, uneventful delivery to primi is brought from delivery room with breathing difficulty. How do you approach and stabilize this newborn?

Task:
- Examine the patient with temperature, airway, breathing, circulation, coma, convulsion and dehydration (TABCD) approach
- Identify the problem and give differential diagnosis
- Lay down priorities in management
- You are not required to take history of the patient

Duration: 10 minutes

Step	***Tick here***
Basics: • Wash hands, ensure asepsis as required • Introduce self and role • Confirm patient identity • Explain you are here to examine • Gain consent from care giver	
Are there any *"life-threatening"* sign *PROMPT:* No life-threatening signs present *Concludes:* I shall proceed to further assessment	
Thermal assessment: *Ask:* What is the baby temperature? *PROMPT:* The temperature is 36°C *Concludes:* Identifies hypothermia	
Action: Ensures baby is kept under warmer on skin probe set at 36.5°C	
Airway assessment: *Ask:* • Is there spontaneous breathing and visible secretions • Any audible sounds *PROMPT:* Baby is breathing normally, cries, and there are no visible secretions *Concludes:* Babies airway is patent *Action:* Ensure "sniffing position"	

Contd...

Contd...

Step	*Tick here*
Breathing assessment: *Ask:* • What is the respiratory rate, chest retractions, air entry, and breath sounds • How is the mental status • What is the reading on pulse oximeter *PROMPT:* Breathing is spontaneous with intercostal indrawing and intermittent grunt. Oxygen saturation (SpO_2) is 88%. *Concludes:* Identifies moderate respiratory distress with hypoxia. *Action:* Monitor with pulse oximetry. Ensure temperature is 36.5°C. Does a quick oral suction. Keeps baby in "sniffing position". Asks to reassess every few minutes.	
Circulatory assessment: *Ask:* • What is the heart rate (HR), peripheral pulses, color, capillary refill time (CRT), and skin temperature • How is the mental status • What is the blood pressure (BP) and urine output *PROMPT:* HR is 150 beats/min, pulses are well felt, color is pale pink. CRT is instant. Baby cries in between. BP is not available. Urine passed in delivery room. *Concludes:* Circulation is fair.	
Dextrose assessment: *Ask:* What is the Glucostix *PROMPT:* Glucostix is 40 mg% *Concludes:* Identifies normoglycemia.	
Problem identification: • This is a preterm, low birth weight (LBW), with moderate respiratory distress with hypoxia • The baby has stable temperature, airway, and circulation • Cause of respiratory distress is most probably respiratory distress syndrome (RDS).	
Plan of action: • Hospitalize and stabilize under warmer • Place baby on a multichannel monitor • Secure intravenous (IV) line. Collect blood culture to rule out sepsis. • Consider starting continuous positive airway pressure (CPAP) at flow of 5 liters per minute ensuring consistent bubbling, positive end-expiratory pressure (PEEP) of 5 cmH_2O ensuring no chest retraction, fraction of inspired oxygen (FiO_2) of 0.5 with target SpO_2 of 91–95% • Monitor Silverman Anderson Score periodically • Reassess by next 30 minutes for need for surfactant • Counsel parents and take details of history with special emphasis on antenatal steroids	

CHAPTER

4.1B

Shock

Case: B/o Misha, term, 2.8 kg, uneventful delivery to primi is brought at 20 hours of age with breathing difficulty and poor activity. How do you approach and stabilize this newborn?

Task:
- Examine the patient with temperature, airway, breathing, circulation, coma, convulsion, and dehydration (TABCD) approach
- Identify the problem and give differential diagnosis
- Lay down priorities in management
- You are *not* required to take history of the patient

Duration: 10 minutes

Step	*Tick here*
Basics: • Wash hands, ensure asepsis as required • Introduce self and role • Confirm patient identity • Explain you are here to examine • Gain consent from care giver	
Are there any *"life-threatening"* signs? *PROMPT:* No life-threatening signs present *Concludes:* I shall proceed to further assessment	
Thermal assessment: *Ask:* What is the baby temperature? *PROMPT:* The temperature is 36°C *Concludes:* Identifies hypothermia	
Action: Ensures baby is kept under warmer on skin probe set at 36.5°C	
Airway assessment: *Ask:* • Is there spontaneous breathing and visible secretions? • Any audible sounds? *PROMPT:* Baby is breathing normally, cries, and there are no visible secretions *Concludes:* Babies airway is patent *Action:* Ensure "sniffing position"	

Contd...

Contd...

Step	*Tick here*
Breathing assessment: *Ask:* • What is the respiratory rate, chest retractions, air entry, and breath sounds? • How is the mental status? • What is the reading on pulse oximeter? *PROMPT:* Breathing is spontaneous with subcostal indrawing and intermittent grunt. Oxygen saturation (SpO_2) is 88% *Concludes:* Identifies mild respiratory distress with hypoxia *Action:* Monitor with pulse oximetry. Ensure temperature is 36.5°C. Does a quick oral suction. Keeps baby in "sniffing position". Asks to reassess every few minutes	
Circulatory assessment: *Ask:* • What is the heart rate (HR), peripheral pulses, color, capillary refill time (CRT), and skin temperature? • How is the mental status? • What is the blood pressure (BP) and urine output? *PROMPT:* HR is 180 beats/min, pulses are weak but felt, skin appears cold, color is pale pink. CRT is 4 seconds. Baby cries in between. BP is 40 systolic. Urine passed at home. *Concludes:* Signs of poor perfusion with hypotension	
Dextrose assessment: *Ask:* What is the Glucostix? *PROMPT:* Glucostix is 40 mg%. *Concludes:* Identifies normoglycemia.	
Problem identification: • This is a term baby, 20 hours old with hypothermia, mild respiratory distress with hypoxia with hypotensive shock on admission. • Cause of hypotensive shock may be sepsis and critical congenital heart disease	
Plan of action: • Hospitalize and stabilize under warmer • Place baby on a multichannel monitor • Secure intravenous (IV) line. Collect blood culture, electrolytes, and arterial blood gas (ABG). • Consider starting nasal oxygen at flow of 1 to 2 liters/min with target SpO_2 of 91–95%. • Give a push of 10 cc/kg of normal saline. Consider point-of-care ultrasound (POCUS), and X-ray chest. • Reassess periodically for need for inotrope. • Counsel parents and take details of history.	

CHAPTER

4.1C

Hypoglycemia

Case: B/o Asha, term, 2 kg, uneventful delivery to primi is brought for poor feeding at 26 hours of age. How do you approach and stabilize this newborn?

Task:

- Examine the patient with temperature, airway, breathing, circulation, coma, convulsion, and dehydration (TABCD) approach
- Identify the problem and give differential diagnosis
- Lay down priorities in management
- You are *not* required to take history of the patient

Duration: 10 minutes

Step	***Tick here***
Basics: • Wash hands, ensure asepsis as required • Introduce self and role • Confirm patient identity • Explain you are here to examine • Gain consent from care giver	
Are there any *"life-threatening"* signs? *PROMPT:* No life-threatening signs present *Concludes:* I shall proceed for further assessment	
Thermal assessment: *Ask:* What is the baby temperature? *PROMPT:* The temperature is normal *Action:* Ensure skin temperature of 36.5°C	
Airway assessment: *Ask:* • Is there spontaneous breathing and visible secretions? • Any audible sounds? *PROMPT:* Baby is breathing normally, cries, and there are no visible secretions *Concludes:* Airway is patent. Shall ensure "sniffing position"	

Contd...

Contd...

Step	*Tick here*
Breathing assessment: *Ask:* • What is the respiratory rate (RR), chest retractions, air entry, and breath sounds? • How is the mental status? • What is recording on pulse oximeter? *PROMPT:* Breathing is spontaneous with no audible sounds or chest indrawing. Oxygen saturation (SpO_2) is 94% *Concludes:* Respiration is normal	
Circulatory assessment: *Ask:* • What is the heart rate (HR), peripheral pulses, color, capillary refill time (CRT), skin temperature? • How is the mental status? • What is the blood pressure (BP) and urine output? *Action:* Fluid bolus, inotropes, monitor BP, and consider point-of-care ultrasound (POCUS) *PROMPT:* The heart rate (HR) is regular at 140 beats/min, pulses well felt, color pink, CRT is 2 seconds, and baby is drowsy but arousable *Concludes:* Stable circulation in a drowsy baby	
Dextrose assessment: *Ask:* How is the Glucostix? *PROMPT:* Glucostix is 35 mg% *Concludes:* This suggests hypoglycemia	
Problem identification: • For 26 hours of age this Glucostix is low s/o hypoglycemia • The infant is symptomatic as there is poor feeding but has stable temperature, airway, breathing, and circulation • Cause of hypoglycemia is most probably inadequate nutritional intake by primi in term intrauterine growth restriction (IUGR) baby with unsupervised feeding and care	
Plan of action: • Hospitalize and stabilize under warmer • Continuously monitor temperature, HR, RR, SpO_2, BP, and urine output • Secure intravenous (IV) line. Collect blood for glucose in fluoride bulb for confirmation. Collect blood culture to rule out sepsis • Give 2 cc/kg 10% glucose push • Start glucose infusion rate (GIR) at 6 to 8 mg/kg/min • Reassess Glucostix 30 minutes later • Counsel parents and take details of history	

CHAPTER 4.2

Breastfeeding

1.

a. Name four components of breastfeeding position that are visible in this picture?

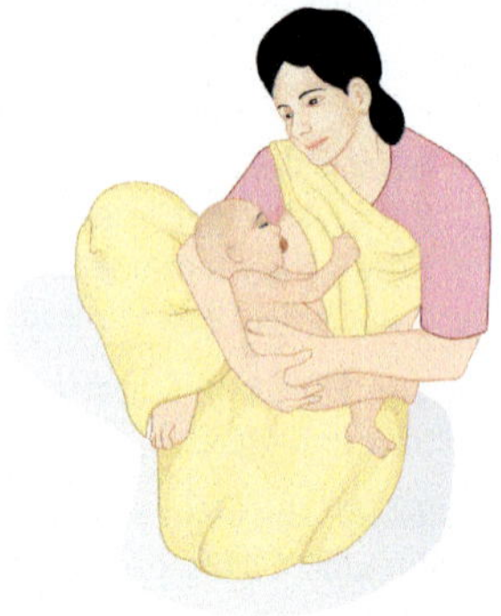

Ans.

The components of breastfeeding position seen in this picture are:

- Neck is straight
- Body is close to mothers body
- Body turned toward mothers
- Whole body supported
- Eye contact between mother and baby

2.

a. Identify the correct latch from the picture.

b. Name four components of a good latch.

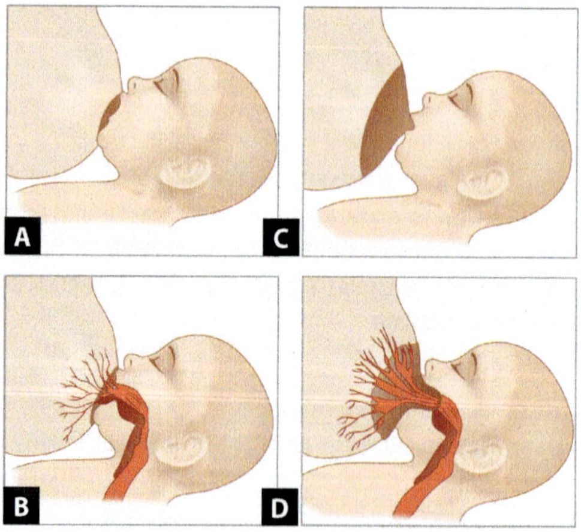

Ans.

a. A

b. Chin touching the breast, wide open mouth, more areola visible above than below, low lip turned outward, and no pain

3. Match the breastfeeding positions and the correct infant need.

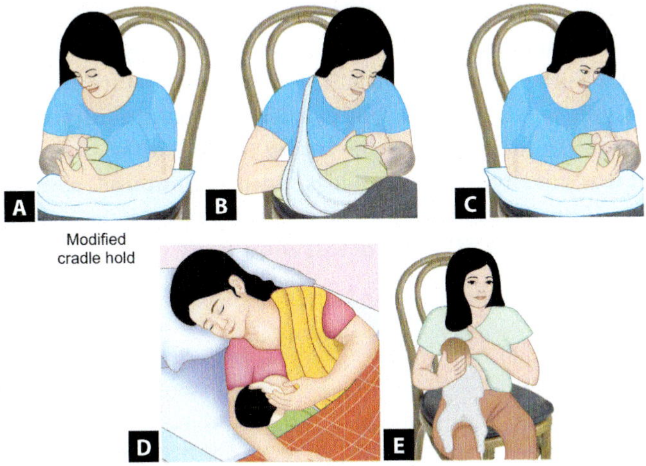

1. Spastic cerebral palsy
2. Floppy infant
3. Preterm infant
4. Cleft palate
5. C-section baby

Ans.

A-2, B-1, C-3, D-5, E-4

4.

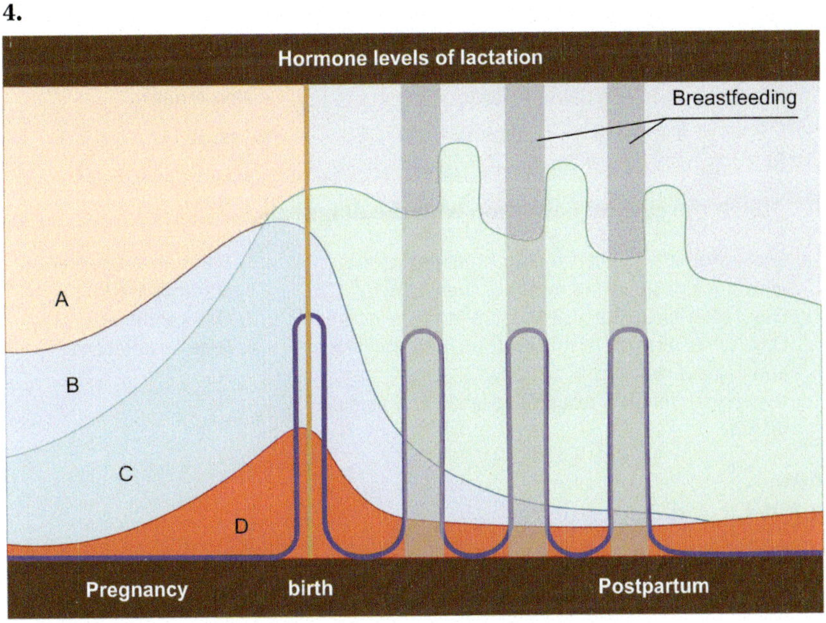

a. Identify the hormone from the picture (A, B, C, D).

Ans.

(a) Progesterone, (b) Prolactin, (c) Oxytocin, (d) Estrogen

5. A preterm neonate born at 30 weeks of gestation ready for discharge after 4 weeks. Nurse wanted to initiate breastfeeding before discharge. Mother's nipple was a little flat but everted after stimulation. Breast was nontender to touch. Baby was trying to suck after stimulation however it was not rhythmic. Mother is requiring minimal assistance for feeding. What is the latch, audible swallowing, type of nipple, comfort and hold (LATCH) score of this condition?

Ans. The LATCH score in this condition is thus 7.

Latch Score				
	0	*1*	*2*	*Total*
L Latch	Too sleepy or reluctant	• Repeated attempts for sustained latch or suck • Hold nipple in mouth • Stimulate to suck	• Grasps breast • Lips flanged • Rhythmic sucking	1
A Audible swallowing	None	A few with stimulation	• Spontaneous and intermittent • Spontaneous and frequent	1
T Type of nipple	Inverted	Flat	Everted after stimulation	2
C Comfort	• Engorged • Severe pain	• Filling • Red	• Soft • Non-tender	2
H Hold	Full assist	Minimal assist	No assist	1

6. Match the clinical condition with the diagnosis.

a. Loose stools, frequent feeding, stool reducing substance positive and mother's breast are full	1. Breast engorgement
b. Day 3 after birth, not able to latch but breasts are full	2. Foremilk feeding
c. Day 7 after birth, poor milk output, maternal fever, and vaginal spotting	3. Oral candidiasis
d. Aversion to feeding, not able to latch, and pain on feeding	4. Retained placenta

Ans.

a-2, b-1, c-4, d-3

CHAPTER 4.3

Respiratory Distress Scoring

CASE 1

A preterm male neonate with birth weight of 1,400 g and 30 weeks of gestation is born to primigravida mother by cesarean section (Indication: Severe preeclampsia). The mother received complete course of antenatal steroids and magnesium sulfate before delivery. The infant has Apgar score of 7/8/8 at 1, 5, and 10 minutes, respectively. The infant developed respiratory distress immediately after birth and was started on T-piece with blended oxygen. The infant was shifted to nursery and the vitals of the infant were:

- Heart rate 148 beats/min
- Respiratory rate 68 breaths/min
- Audible grunting without stethoscope
- Cyanosis on fraction of inspired oxygen (FiO_2) 40%
- Barely audible bilateral air entry
- Upper chest having respiratory lag
- Minimal lower chest retraction
- Minimal xiphoid retraction
- Marked nasal flaring

Questions:

1. Which scoring system to be used to assess severity of respiratory distress?
2. What is the severity score of respiratory distress?
3. Can we use Silverman Andersen Score (SAS) for term infants?
4. What is the importance of severity score in management of infant?

Answers:

1. As the index infant is premature baby we will use SAS because:
    - Tells better about the functional residual capacity (FRC) of lung in case of respiratory distress syndrome (RDS)
    - Assessing decrease in air entry (component of Downes score) in premature infants is difficult as they have very small chest.
2. The SAS of this infant is 7/10. The various components of the scoring system are:

Features	*0*	*1*	*2*	*Index case*
Upper chest movements	None	Respiratory lag	Seesaw respiration	1
Lower chest retractions	None	Minimal	Marked	1
Xiphoid retractions	None	Minimal	Marked	1
Nasal flaring	None	Minimal	Marked	2
Grunting	None	Audible with stethoscope	Audible without stethoscope	2

Examine the infant from side of the warmer and draw an imaginary midaxillary line and the chest anterior to the line is upper chest and below the line is lower chest. Always use the stethoscope for auscultation of grunting if there is no audible grunting.

3. The SAS can be used both in preterm and term infants but it is better to avoid using Downes score in preterm infants.
4. The importance of severity score in management are:
   - Useful as a criteria for initiation of respiratory support (noninvasive) in newborns at a score of ≥3
   - A score of less than 4 indicates mild respiratory distress, 4–7 indicates rmoderate espiratory distress, and more than 7 indicates severe respiratory distress.
   - Objective way to assess the severity of respiratory distress
   - Monitoring of score at regular intervals tells us about improvement or deterioration of the respiratory distress

CASE 2

A term female infant is born with birth weight of 3,240 g and 39 weeks of gestation to a primigravida mother by cesarean section (Indication: Fetal distress with meconium-stained amniotic fluid).

The infant is vigorous and is given an Apgar score of 8/9/9 at 1, 5, and 10 minutes, respectively. The infant developed respiratory distress immediately after birth and was started on T-piece with blended oxygen keeping targeted saturation as goal. The infant was shifted to nursery and the vitals of the infant were:

- Heart rate 156 beats/min
- Respiratory rate 74 breaths/min
- Capillary refill time <3 second
- Audible grunting with stethoscope
- Cyanosis on FiO_2 50%
- Barely audible bilateral air entry
- Upper chest having respiratory lag

- Minimal lower chest retraction
- Minimal xiphoid retraction
- Marked nasal flaring

Questions:

1. Which scoring system to be used to assess severity of respiratory distress?
2. What is the severity score of respiratory distress?

Answers:

1. We can use both SAS and Downes score for assessment of severity of respiratory distress in this case. In term infants, Downes score is preferred as it tells about the oxygen requirement by the infant, hence telling severity of parenchymal disease.
2. The SAS of the infant is 7. The Downes score of the infant is 8. The various components of Downes score are:

Features	***0***	***1***	***2***	***Index case***
Cyanosis	None	In room air	In 40% FiO_2	2
Retractions	None	Mild	Severe	1
Air entry	Normal	Decreased	Barely audible	2
Grunting	None	Audible with stethoscope	Audible without stethoscope	2
Respiratory rates (per minute)	<60	60–80	>80 or apnea	1

A score of less than 4 indicates no or mild respiratory distress, 4–7 indicates rmoderate espiratory distress, and more than 7 indicates severe respiratory distress.

Note:

- If infant is on invasive ventilation, the maximum score of each scoring system will be 8 as these infants will not be having grunting, as glottis remains open because of endotracheal tube.
- If infant is on continuous positive airway pressure (CPAP), the maximum SAS will be 8 as it is not possible to see nasal flaring in these infants.

CHAPTER

4.4 Arterial Blood Gas

1.

pH	7.31	S	Electrolytes	a. Interpret the arterial blood gas (ABG).
PaO_2	99 mm Hg	Na	140 mEq/L	b. Name four common etiologies for this ABG.
PCO_2	26 mm Hg	K	5 mEq/L	c. Calculate the anion gap.
HCO_3	12 mEq/L	Cl	100 mEq/L	d. Calculate the alveolar-arterial oxygen gradient (AaO_2) gradient with fraction of inspired oxygen (FiO_2) 0.5%
				e. What ventilator setting would you change—peak inspiratory pressure (PIP), positive end-expiratory pressure (PEEP), and FiO_2?
				f. Name two conditions with normal anion gap acidosis.
				g. What is the compensation formula in this case?

Ans.

a. Metabolic acidosis with hyperoxia.

b. Hypoxia, sepsis, shock, acute renal failure, anemia, hypoglycemia, hypothermia, patent ductus arteriosus (PDA), and inborn error of metabolism.

c. $140 - (100 + 12) = 28$. Anion gap is high.

d. $(760 - 45) \times 0.5 - 26 = 331$.

e. Treat the cause of metabolic acidosis as this is secondary respiratory alkalosis.

f. Renal tubular acidosis, extreme prematurity, and drug (acetazolamide).

g. $[(1.5 \times HCO_3^-) + 8 \pm 2]$

2.

pH	7.09	S	Electrolytes	a. Interpret the ABG.
PaO_2	126 mm Hg	Na	140 mEq/L	b. Calculate the AaO_2 gradient, a/A and respiratory index with FiO_2 0.6%.
PCO_2	54 mm Hg	K	5 mEq/L	c. What immediate action would you take?
HCO_3	16 mEq/L	Cl	100 mEq/L	d. What is the impact of CO_2 retention on lungs and brain?
SpO_2	98%			e. What are the target saturations for babies on respiratory support?

Ans.

a. Acute respiratory acidosis with metabolic acidosis.
b. 239, 0.5, and 1.8
c. Evaluate for respiratory efforts and do a transillumination to rule out pneumothorax. Mechanical ventilation if efforts are poor.
d. Increased pulmonary vascular resistance and intraventricular hemorrhage (IVH) (increased blood flow to brain).
e. 91–95%

3.

pH	7.45	S	Electrolytes
PaO_2	114 mm Hg	Na	130 mEq/L
PCO_2	28 mm Hg	K	4.5 mEq/L
HCO_3	20 mEq/L	Cl	110 mEq/L

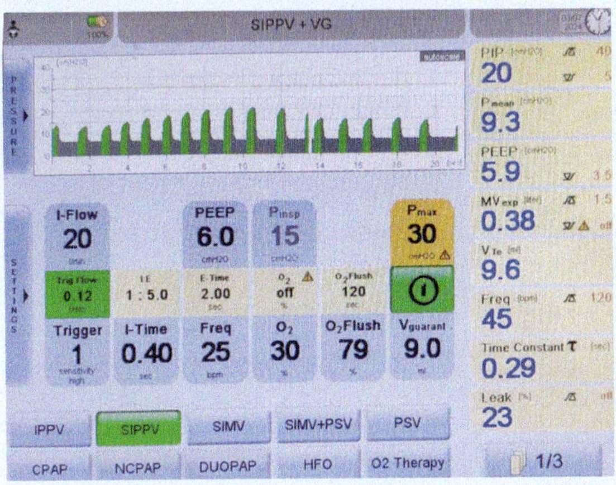

a. Interpret the ABG.
b. Calculate the OI, RI, and OSI.
c. What immediate action would you take?
d. What is the impact of CO_2 washout?
e. At what leak volume guarantee is not advisable?

(OI: oxygenation index; OSI: oxygen saturation index; RI: respiratory index)

Ans.

a. Respiratory alkalosis with hyperoxia.
b. 2.44, 0.5, and 2.84.
c. Reduce the PIP.
d. Increased risk of periventricular leukomalacia (PVL), deafness, and cognitive delay.
e. 40% if not leak adjustment is done by the ventilator.

4.

pH	7.20	S	Electrolytes
PaO_2	90 mm Hg	Na	140 mEq/L
PCO_2	18 mm Hg	K	7.5 mEq/L
HCO_3	10 mEq/L	Cl	100 mEq/L

a. Interpret the ABG.
b. Name four potential problems with sodabicarb therapy.
c. What are the two causes of severe metabolic acidosis with hyperammonemia?
d. What is the most likely cause of this?

Ans.

a. Metabolic acidosis with respiratory compensation with hyperoxia.
b. Shifts the oxygen dissociation curve to the left causing O_2 retention, CO_2 builds up taking away the respiratory drive, precipitates IVH or acute renal failure due to hyperosmolar solution, and skin extravasation injury.
c. Organic acidemia and pyruvate dehydrogenase deficiency.
d. Congenital adrenal hyperplasia as there is acidosis, hypernatremia, and hyperkalemia.

5.

pH	7.38	S	Electrolytes	a. Interpret the ABG.
PaO_2	75 mm Hg	Na	140 mEq/L	b. Which single ventilator knob you will change?
PCO_2	65 mm Hg	K	5 mEq/L	c. What is the effect of air bubble on gases?
HCO_3	35 mEq/L	Cl	100 mEq/L	d. What is the effect of delayed sample processing on the gases?
				e. What is the effect of cry during sample collection?

Ans.

a. Chronic respiratory acidosis with metabolic alkalosis with hyperoxia.
b. Decrease the PEEP.
c. Increases PaO_2 and decreases PCO_2.
d. Increases PCO_2 and decreases PaO_2.
e. Decreases PaO_2 and PCO_2.

CHAPTER

4.5

Clinical Spots

1.

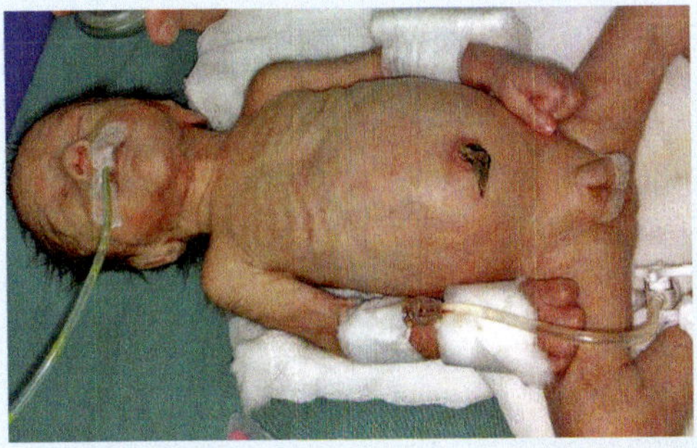

a. Identify three clinical signs in this preterm.
b. Name two primary risk factors for this condition.
c. Name two complications you would anticipate.
d. What classical findings on X-ray abdomen confirm the diagnosis?
e. Name a poor prognostic sign on X-ray.

Ans.

a. Tense distended abdomen, erythema of abdominal wall, and significant gastric residues.
b. Prematurity, formula feeds, and sepsis.
c. Perforation, peritonitis, sepsis, and shock.
d. Pneumatosis intestinalis—visualization of small amounts of air within the bowel wall
e. Presence of portal venous gas

2.

Day 5, term, 2.8 kg, vacuum delivery, admitted for seizures. Cerebrospinal fluid (CSF) done as follows:

CSF	***Day 5***
Glucose	10
Proteins	550
Cells	3,600

a. What is the gold standard for confirmation of your diagnosis?
b. Name two acute complications.
c. Name two chronic complications.
d. Name two vascular complications.

Ans.

a. CSF culture.
b. Cerebral edema, increased intracranial pressure (ICP), ventriculitis, cerebritis, and cerebral infarction.

c. Hydrocephalus, brain abscess, and subdural effusion.
d. Cerebral venous thrombosis and arterial stroke.

3. Day 10, home delivery, term, 2.3 kg, admitted with fever since 1 day, poor feeding since 12 hours. Exclusive breastfed. Awake, alert with stable vital parameters. Rooting present. Sucking absent. Startles to noise or touch. Develops arching of back intermittently.

a. What is the clinical diagnosis?
b. Name three common risk factors for this condition.
c. What is the drug of choice?
d. Name two anticipated complications?

Ans.

a. Neonatal tetanus.
b. Unvaccinated mother, home delivery, septic cutting of umbilical cord, application of dung or mud, etc., to cord.
c. Tetanus immunoglobulin.
d. Vocal cord palsy leading to respiratory distress, autonomic dysfunction, paralytic ileus, aspiration, urine retention, and seizures.

4.

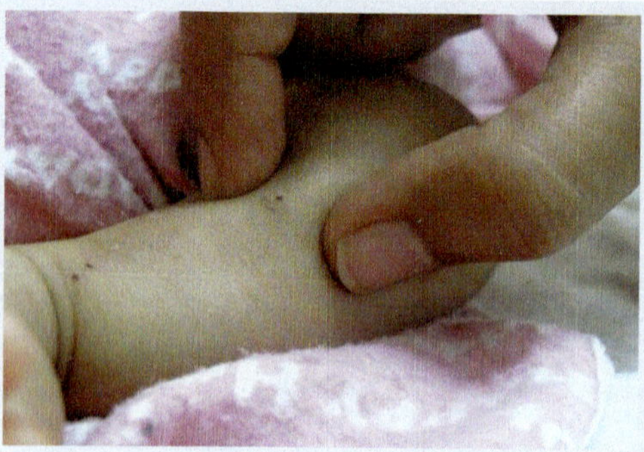

Day 4, term, baby has poor feeding, cry, activity, and breathing. There is moaning, diffuse woody to stony hard induration of extremities, nonpitting, nonpinchable, with reduced joint mobility. Associated shock and cold extremities are noted.

a. What is the clinical sign?
b. Name two sites where the changes are absent.
c. Name the closest mimicking skin condition.
d. Name two histologic findings in this condition.

Ans.

a. Sclerema.
b. Genitals, palms, and soles.
c. Subcutaneous fat necrosis and scleredema.
d. Necrosis of subcutaneous fat tissue, needle-shaped cleft formation within fat cells, thick fibrosis surrounding fat lobules, and minimal inflammatory infiltration, no granulomatous changes.

5.

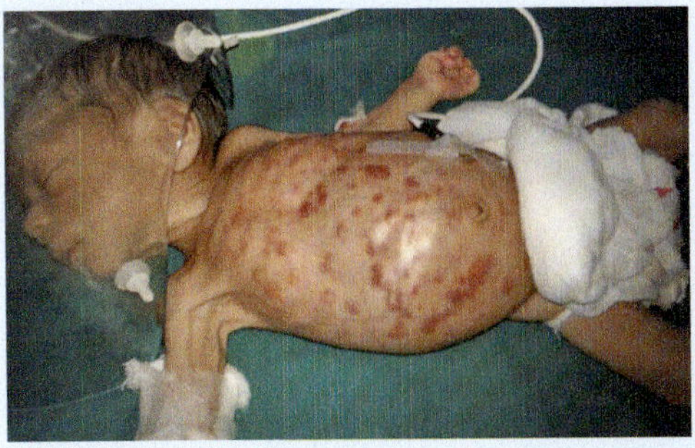

a. Identify the skin lesion.
b. What does the histopathology signify?
c. Name two hematological causes.
d. Name two neoplastic causes.

Ans.

a. Blue berry muffin rash.
b. Dermal erythropoiesis.
c. Twin-to-twin transfusion syndrome, hereditary spherocytosis, and hemolytic disease of the newborn.
d. Mastocytosis, histiocytosis, neuroblastoma, rhabdomyosarcoma, and leukemia.

6.

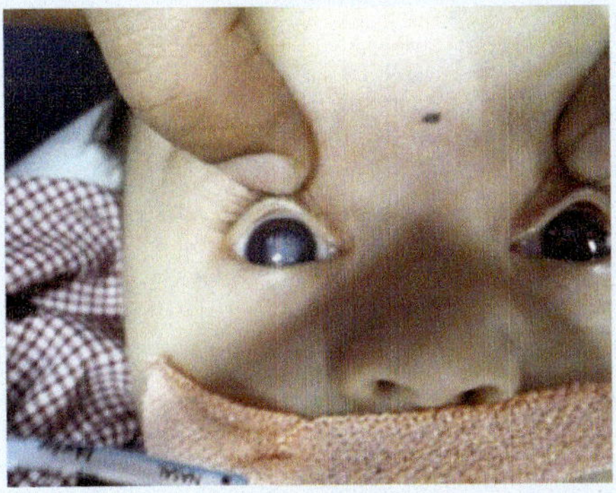

a. Name four causes of leukocoria.
b. Name a screening test to pick this problem in normal newborn.
c. Presence of failure to thrive and vomiting should raise suspicion of which disorder in this baby?
d. What is the ideal time to operate congenital cataract?
e. What is the most common complication of congenital cataract surgery?
f. What is the most common inheritance of congenital cataract?

Ans.

a. Cataract, glaucoma, retinopathy of prematurity (ROP), retinoblastoma, persistent fetal vasculature, and trauma.
b. Red reflex test by direct ophthalmoscope.
c. Galactosemia.
d. 6–8 weeks.
e. Glaucoma.
f. Autosomal dominant.

7.

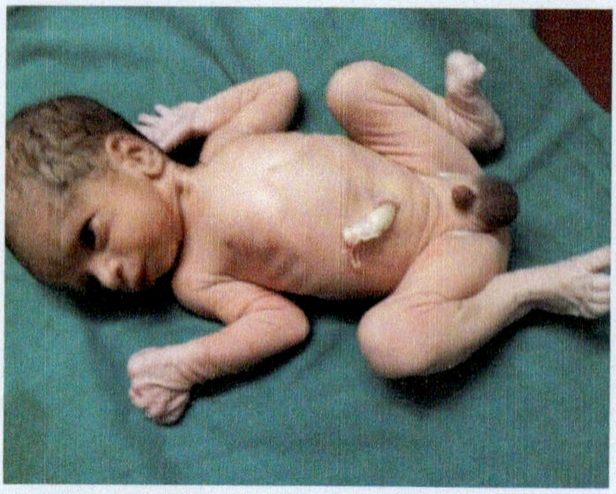

Term, 2.2 kg at birth:

a. What is the diagnosis?
b. Name two problems you anticipate in the delivery room.
c. Name two interventions you should do at birth in all such well babies.
d. How does fundal height during pregnancy give clue to possibility of fetal growth restriction?
e. Name the components of biophysical profile.
f. Name four problems you anticipate in first 48 hours.
g. Which babies should be subjected to genetic testing?
h. What therapy should be offered for persistent short stature at 3–4 years of age?

Ans.

a. Small for gestational age (SGA).
b. Hypothermia, asphyxia, meconium aspiration, and congenital anomaly.
c. Early skin-to-skin contact and early exclusive breastfeeding.
d. Fundal height at least 3 cm less than the gestational age in weeks.
e. Nonstress test heart rate monitoring, fetal breathing movement, gross fetal movement, fetal tone, and amniotic fluid volume.
f. Hypoglycemia, hypoxic ischemic encephalopathy, jaundice, polycythemia, poor feeding, and hypocalcemia
g. Presence of dysmorphic features, major malformations, microcephaly, and skeletal abnormality.
h. Growth hormone therapy.

8.

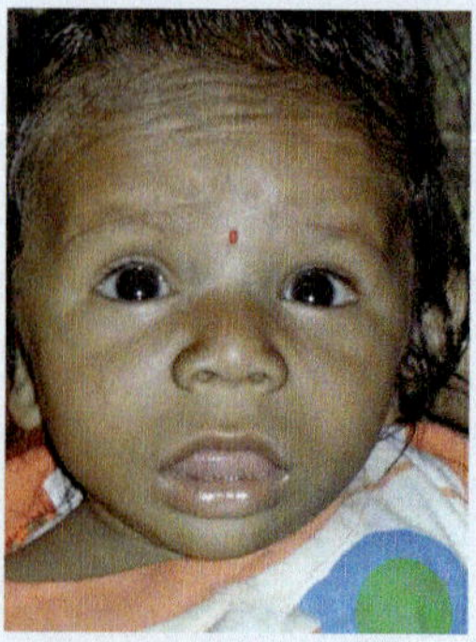

a. What screening test can prevent this abnormality?
b. What is the most common cause of this condition?
c. Why are these babies normal at birth or in early neonatal period?
d. Name conditions where repeat screening is routinely advised irrespective of initial results.
e. Below what age treatment started leads to normal cognition.

Ans.

a. Thyroid-stimulating hormone (TSH) or T4 screen on cord blood or day 3.
b. Thyroid dysgenesis—agenesis, ectopic, or hypoplastic gland.
c. Due to partial maternal thyroxine hormone transfer.
d. Preterm, sick, and multiple births with same sex.
e. Before 2 weeks of age.

9. Interpret

a.
   1. Low T4, high TSH
   2. Normal T4, high TSH
   3. Low T4, normal TSH

b. At what age is trial off therapy recommended to decide transient or permanent hypothyroidism?
c. Name routine medications which interfere with thyroxine absorption.
d. When should thyroid test be done following alteration of thyroxine dose?

Ans.

a. (1) Primary hypothyroidism, (2) Subclinical hypothyroidism, (3) Central hypothyroidism.
b. 36 months age.
c. Iron and calcium.
d. 4–6 weeks.

10.

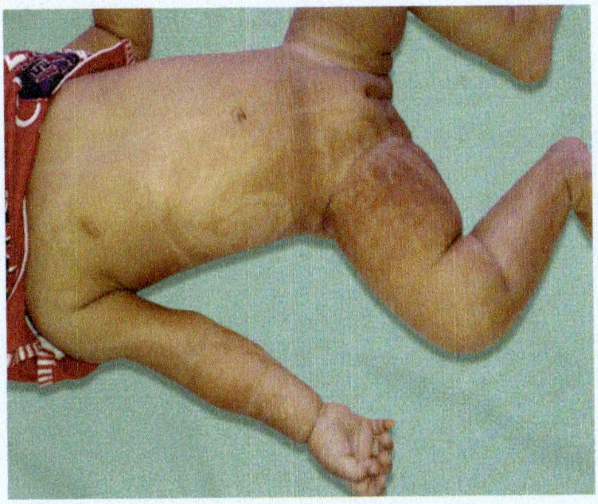

a. Describe the skin lesion.
b. What is the diagnosis?
c. How is the diagnosis confirmed?
d. Name two systems most commonly involved and two problems you would anticipate in future.

Ans.

a. Hypopigmented macules following the lines of Blaschko, arranged in sharply demarcated whorls, streaks, and patches.
b. Hypomelanosis of Ito.
c. Examination under Wood's lamp enhances the hypopigmentation.

d. Central nervous system (CNS) and musculoskeletal. Seizures, psychomotor delay, hemihypertrophy, asymmetric limbs, finger abnormalities, hypotonia, scoliosis, and short stature.

11. Match the characteristics with human pathogens.

Organism	*Characteristics*
1. *Pseudomonas*	a. Obligate anaerobes
2. *Streptococcus, Staphylococcus*	b. Obligate aerobes
3. *Neisseria*	c. Gram positive cocci
4. *Escherichia, Klebsiella, Proteus*	d. Gram negative cocci
	e. Facultative anaerobes
	f. Obligate intracellular parasites

Ans. 1-b, 2-c, 3-d, 4-e

CHAPTER

4.6

X-rays and Scans

1.

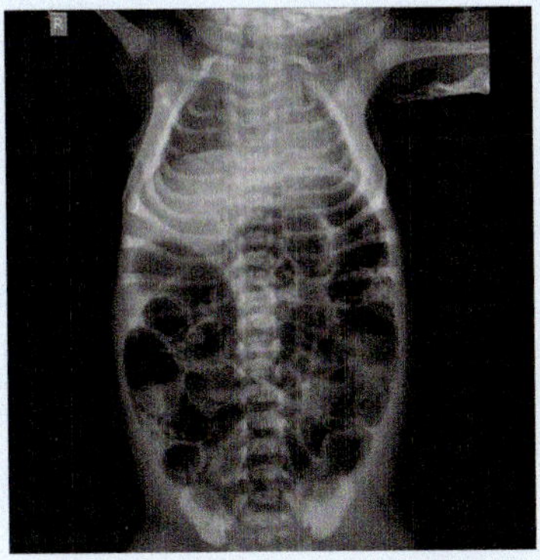

a. Identify the radiologic sign.
b. What classification is used to stage the disease?
c. At what stage of the disease do you consider addition of antibiotics for anaerobes?
d. Name two proven strategies for its prevention.
e. Name a clinical sign to signify return of bowel function.

Ans.

a. Intraluminal air called pneumatosis intestinalis, also called "bangle sign" is seen as curvilinear lucencies adjacent to the intestinal lumen in right upper quadrant.
b. Bell's classification.
c. Stage 2B of Bell's classification.
d. Probiotics, human breast milk, and antenatal steroids.
e. Presence of normal bowel movements.

2.

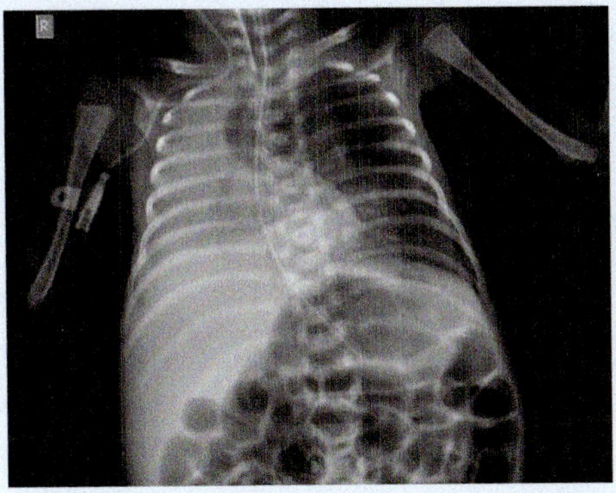

a. Identify two interventions.
b. Identify two lung signs.
c. What is the most common cause for this problem?
d. How would you position the baby?

Ans.

a. Intubation and feeding tube in situ.
b. High endotracheal tube (ETT), collapse of the right lung, and compensatory emphysema of left lung.
c. Blocked right main bronchus due to mucous plug or secretions or lobar emphysema of left lung.
d. Affected side up—left lateral position.

3.

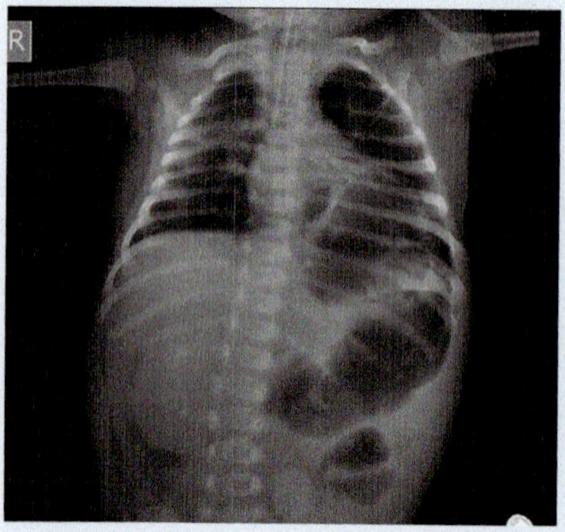

a. Identify two lung signs.
b. Name the most common organism responsible for the lung pathology.
c. Name two differential diagnoses.
d. What is the antibiotic of choice?

Ans.

a. Bilateral perihilar infiltration, right lung more than left, and multiple air filled cavities in left lung.
b. *Staphylococcus aureus.*
c. Congenital diaphragmatic hernia and congenital pulmonary adenomatoid malformation of lung.
d. Vancomycin.

4.

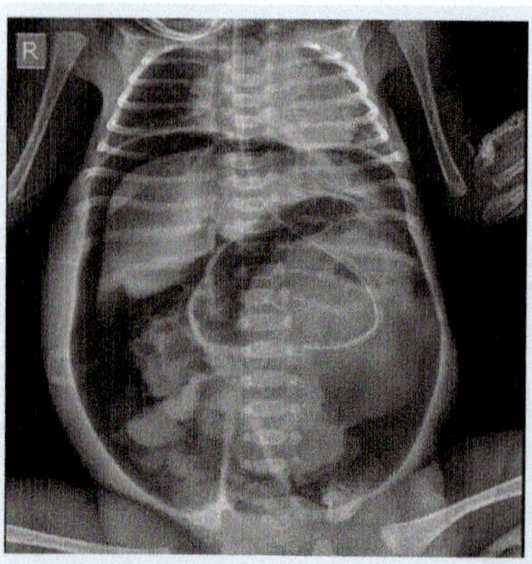

a. Identify the radiologic sign.
b. Name the most common cause for this problem.
c. Name two causes in term infants with this sign.
d. What is the procedure of choice in surgically unfit babies?

Ans.

a. Football sign—shows free air under both domes of diaphragm and in the whole peritoneal cavity.
b. Necrotizing enterocolitis.
c. Malrotation with midgut volvulus and meconium ileus.
d. Peritoneal drain.

5.

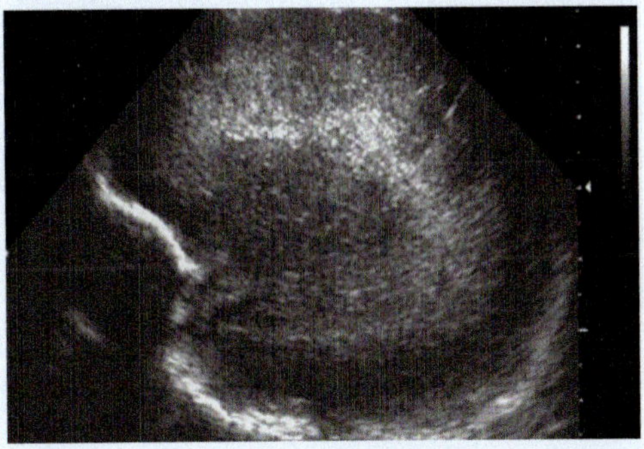

a. Identify the brain scan abnormality.
b. How do you differentiate it from hemorrhage?
c. Name two prenatal risk factors.
d. Name two iatrogenic causes.
e. Babies are at risk for which type of cerebral palsy?
f. Name two squeal in term infants.

Ans.

a. Increased periventricular echogenicity.
b. No mass effect with periventricular leukomalacia (PVL).
c. Chorioamnionitis, preterm premature rupture of membrane (PPROM), placental abruption, and bacterial vaginosis.
d. Hyperventilation, no antenatal steroids, blood pressure (BP) fluctuation, and sepsis.
e. Spastic diplegia.
f. Intellectual disability, epilepsy, and cerebral palsy with cognitive delay with epilepsy.

6.

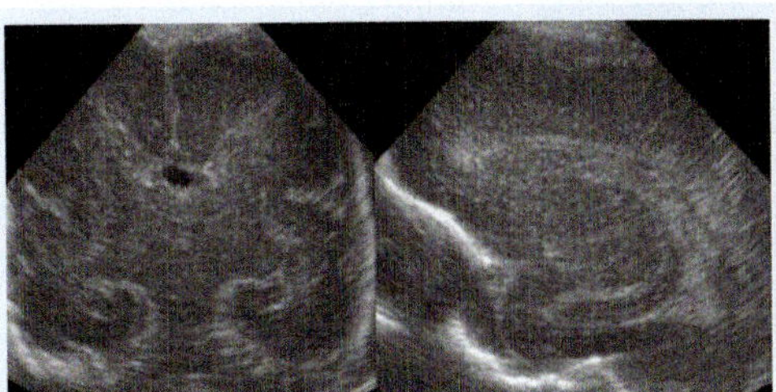

a. Identify the abnormality and severity.
b. Name the only prophylactic postnatal intervention to prevent it.
c. Name two interventions in delivery room which may precipitate the condition.
d. Name two iatrogenic causes.

Ans.

a. Intraventricular hemorrhage—grade 2.
b. Intravenous (IV) indomethacin.

c. Milking of cord, head low position, shaking the baby, sodabicarb bolus, and ventilation with high pressures.
d. Ventilation with high pressures, rapid boluses/infusions, and sodabicarb.

7.

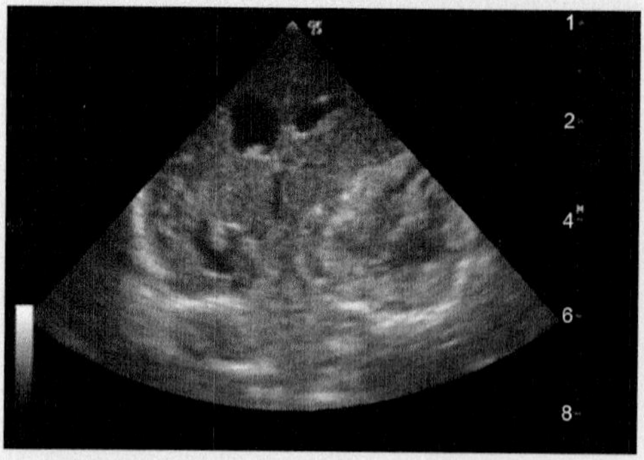

a. Diagnosis.
b. Name a drug to prevent it.
c. Name two maternal predisposing risk factors.
d. Name the most common cause in symptomatic and asymptomatic term infants.
e. Name the most common laboratory abnormality in term infants.

Ans.

a. Massive cerebral hemorrhage.
b. Vitamin K.
c. Cephalopelvic disproportion, prolonged labor, difficult labor, and abnormal presentation.
d. Subarachnoid hemorrhage and subdural hemorrhage.
e. Thrombocytopenia.

8.

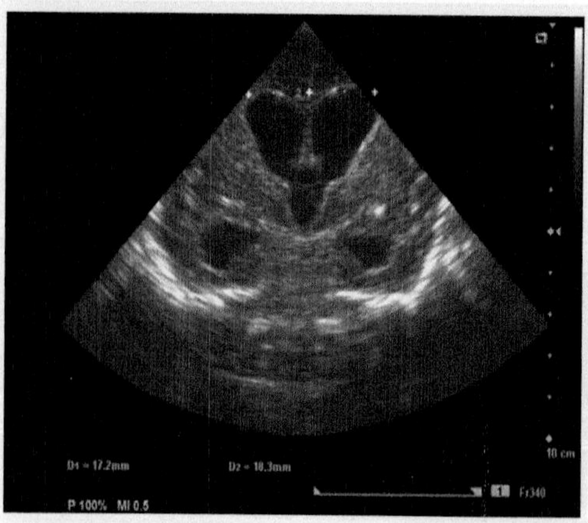

a. What is the diagnosis?
b. Name the most common cause in newborn.
c. Name two causes which work both prenatal and postnatal.
d. Name two maternal drugs predisposing to this condition.
e. Name the most common heritable form.
f. Name a condition with similar appearance but normal intracranial pressure.

Ans.

a. Hydrocephalus.
b. Post hemorrhagic hydrocephalus.
c. Hemorrhage, infection, or neoplasm.
d. Misoprostol, metronidazole, and isotretinoin.

e. X-linked hydrocephalus associated with stenosis of the aqueduct of sylvius (HSAS).
f. "Hydrocephalus ex vacuo", i.e., compensatory enlargement of the cerebral ventricles and/or subarachnoid space due to encephalomalacia and/or periventricular volume loss.

9.

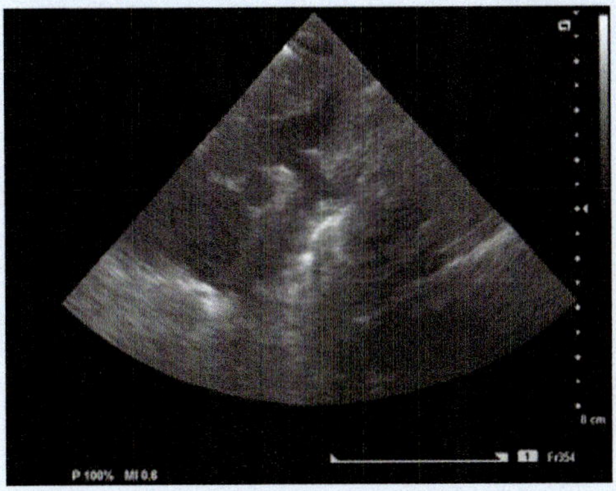

a. What is the diagnosis?
b. Name a clinical clue to diagnose it in well baby.
c. Name lifesaving intervention in neonatal intensive care unit (NICU).
d. Name a screening test to diagnose in normal newborn.
e. What test is recommended in girl child with this condition?

Ans.

a. Coarctation of aorta.
b. Absent femoral pulses, differential blood pressure, and sudden deterioration.
c. Prostaglandin infusion.
d. Pulse oximetry screen at hospital discharge.
e. Karyotyping as Turner syndrome is most commonly associated with it.

10.

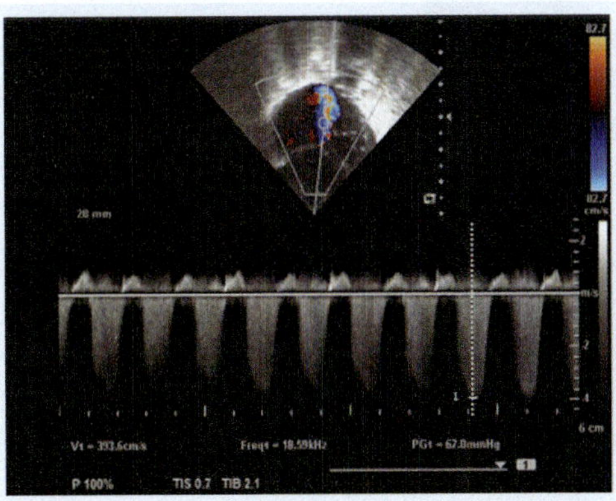

a. Identify the echo parameter.
b. What is it used to measure?
c. Name two conditions which make it technically difficult to measure.
d. Parasternal short-axis view is used for which echo parameter?
e. Which echocardiographic view is used to assess for ductus arteriosus shunt?

Ans.

a. Tricuspid regurgitant (TR) jet velocity.
b. Right ventricular systolic pressure (RVSP).

c. Presence of pulmonary stenosis or a significant ventricular septal defect.
d. Evaluation of interventricular septum (IVS) and left ventricular (LV) size.
e. High left parasternal "ductal" view.

11.

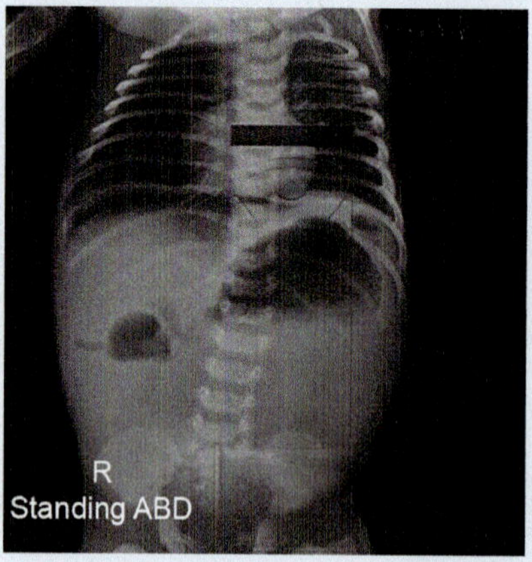

a. Identify the sign.
b. Name four differential diagnoses.
c. What does its prenatal diagnosis signify?
d. What systemic anomaly search would you undertake?

Ans.

a. Double bubble shadow.
b. Duodenal web, duodenal atresia, duodenal stenosis, annular pancreas, and midgut volvulus.
c. Trisomy 21
d. Vertebral defects, anal atresia, cardiac defects, tracheoesophageal fistula, renal anomalies, and limb abnormalities (VACTERL).

12.

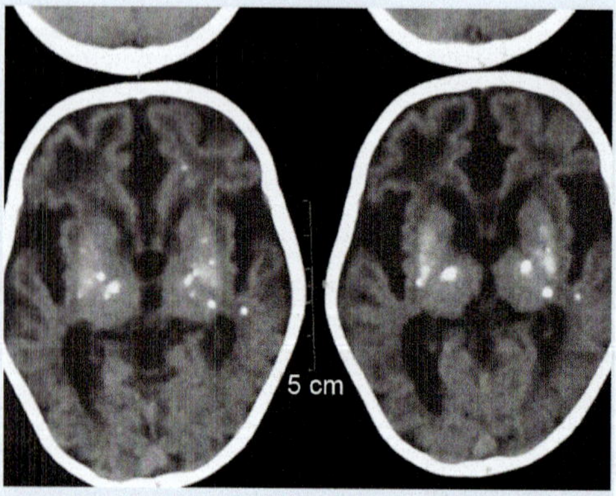

a. Identify the pathology.
b. Name two postnatal causes.
c. Name two conditions with associated cutaneous markers.
d. Why cytomegalovirus (CMV) calcifications are periventricular?
e. Name the triad for congenital toxoplasmosis.

Ans.

a. Periventricular calcification.
b. Bacterial meningitis and ventriculitis.
c. Tuberous sclerosis, Sturge-Weber syndrome.

d. Due to damage to the germinal matrix, which results in white matter atrophy, ventriculomegaly, and abnormalities in neuronal migration.
e. Hydrocephalus, chorioretinitis, and intracranial calcifications.

13.

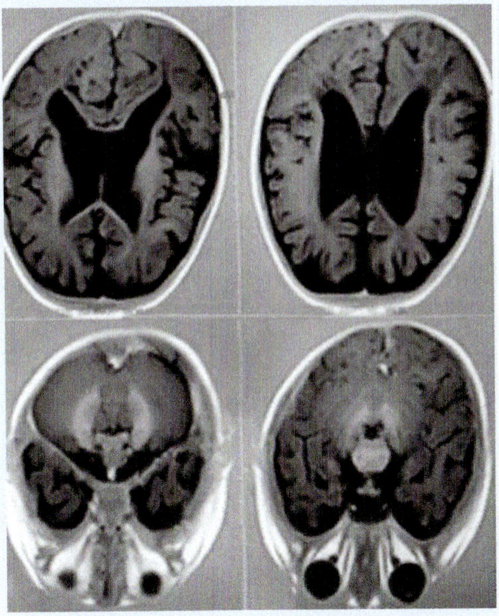

a. Identify the pathology on MRI brain.
b. Name an iatrogenic risk factor.
c. Name an evidence-based intervention to prevent it.
d. Name two perinatal risk factors.
e. Which neonatal reflex remains persistent with this pathology?

Ans.

a. Periventricular leukomalacia.
b. Hyperventilation.
c. Prenatal steroids.
d. Placental abruption and fetal acidosis.
e. Asymmetric tonic neck reflex.

14.

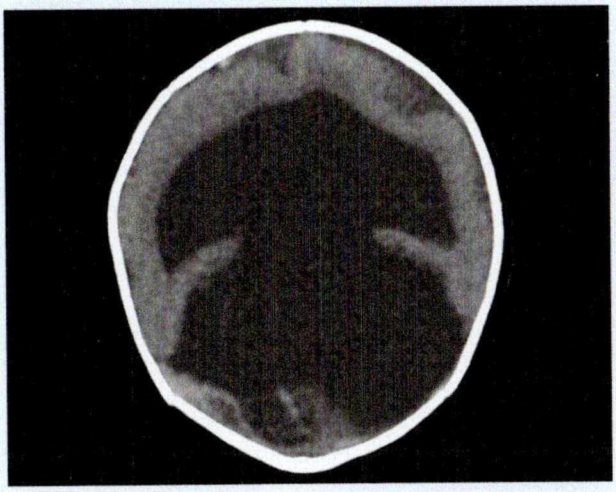

a. What is the diagnosis?
b. Name the most common genetic abnormality associated.
c. Name two midline anomalies associated with it.
d. Name two differential diagnoses.

Ans.

a. Holoprosencephaly—fusion of cerebral hemispheres.
b. Trisomy 13.
c. Cleft lip/palate, ocular hypotelorism, cyclopia, and proboscis.
d. Septo-optic dysplasia, hydranencephaly, porencephalic cyst, and arachnoid cyst.

CHAPTER

4.7

Pulmonary Graphics

1.

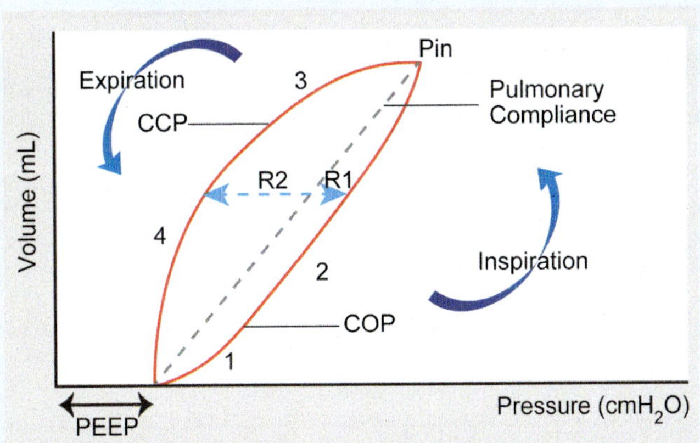

a. What are R1, R2, COP, and CCP?
b. What is the beaking effect and that is the normal C20/C?
c. What ventilation parameters can be adjusted using this graph?
d. What will happen to this graph if the newborns develop hemodynamically significant patent ductus arteriosus (hsPDA)?

Ans.

a. R1 is inspiratory resistance, R2 is expiratory resistance, COP is critical opening pressure, and CCP is critical closing pressure.
b. The last segment of the graph flattening is beaking effect. Normal C20/C is >1.
c. Positive end-expiratory pressure (PEEP) and peak inspiratory pressure (PIP).
d. The graph will become more flat. Compliance will reduce.

2.

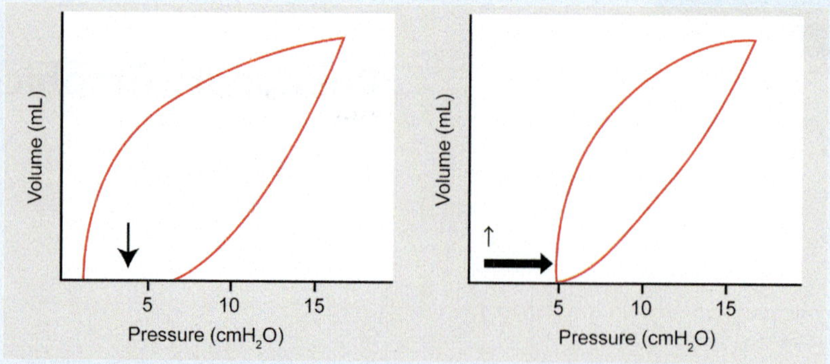

a. What is the problem in the first graph?
b. What ventilation parameter is changed to obtain the second pressure-volume (PV) loop?

Ans.

a. There is significant atelectasis.
b. PEEP is increased to 5 cm from <2 cm.

3.

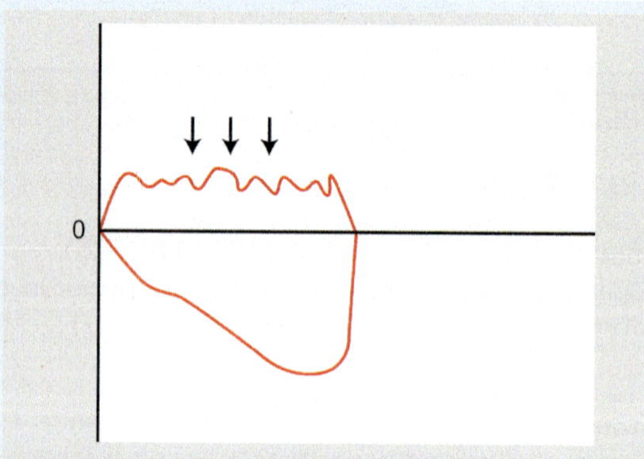

a. Identify the graph.
b. What is the problem in this ventilated newborn?
c. What procedure is required to correct this graph?

Ans.

a. This is flow volume loop.
b. There are secretions in the endotracheal (ET) tube.
c. The baby needs ET suction.

4.

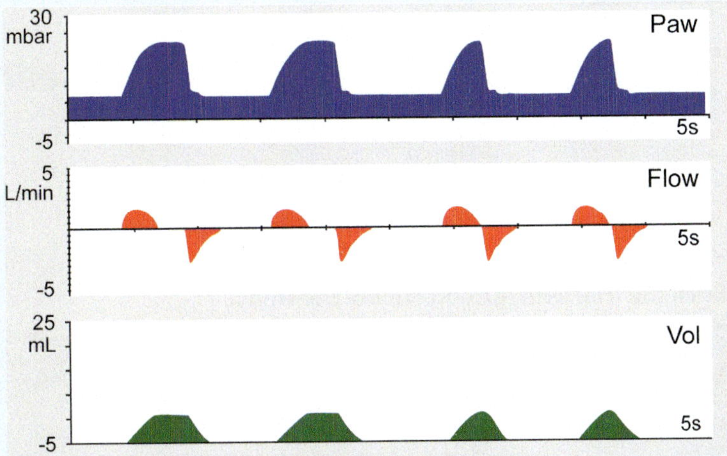

a. Identify the modes of ventilation in this newborn?
b. What is the change in ventilation mode shown here? Explain.

Ans.

a. The first-time waves are of assist control and the second two are of pressure support mode of ventilation.
b. The gap between in the inspiratory and expiratory flows in lost in the last two waves.

5.

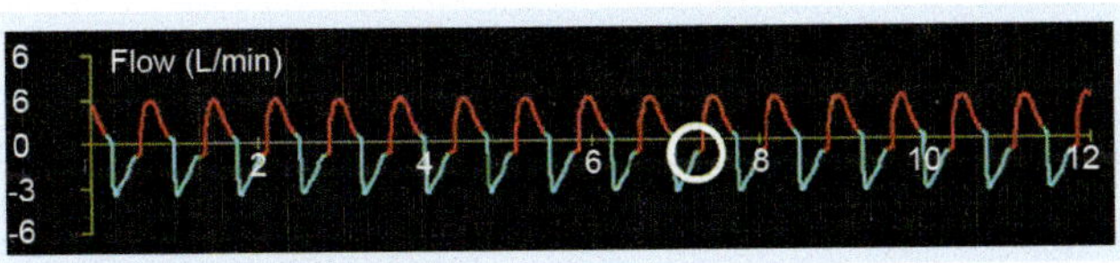

a. What is shown in this graph?
b. How will correct this problem?

Ans.

a. The graph is showing auto PEEP.
b. Increase the expiratory time.

CHAPTER

4.8

Research

1. Match the trial with the objective of the study.

1. TIPP trial
2. SAVE trial
3. SUPPORT trial
4. CAP trial
5. TOP trial
6. COIN trial
7. BOOST trial

a. Caffeine therapy for apnea of prematurity
b. Inhaled nitric oxide for premature infants with severe respiratory failure
c. Early continuous positive airway pressure (CPAP) versus surfactant in extremely preterm infant
d. Higher or lower hemoglobin transfusion thresholds for preterm infants
e. Long-term effects of indomethacin prophylaxis in extremely-low-birth-weight infants
f. Adverse effects of early dexamethasone treatment in extremely-low-birth-weight infants
g. Nasal CPAP or intubation for very preterm infants at birth
h. Outcomes of two trials of oxygen-saturation targets in preterm infants

Ans. 1-e, 2-f, 3-c, 4-a, 5-d, 6-g, 7-h

2.

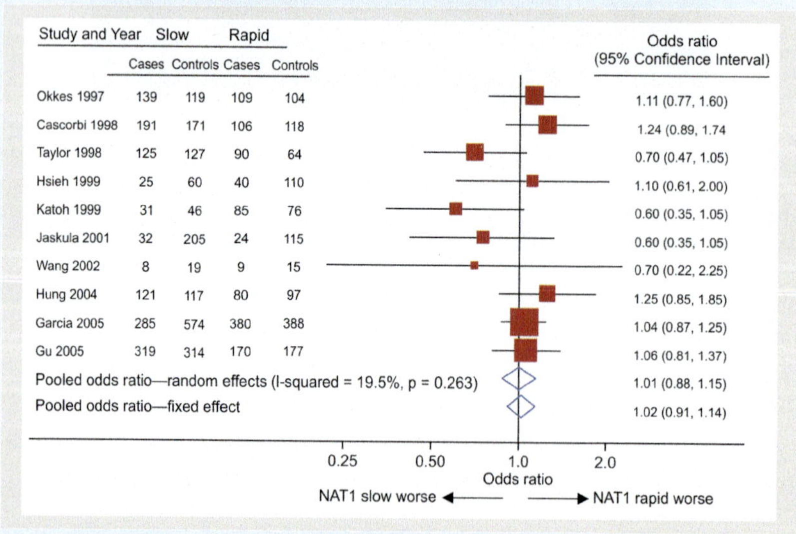

a. Identify the graph.
b. What does the square and area of square represent?
c. What does the horizontal and vertical line represent?
d. What does diamond represent?
e. What does center of diamond represent?

Ans.

a. Forrest plot.
b. Square represents a study in the meta-analysis and area corresponds to the weight of the study in the meta-analysis.
c. Horizontal line through the square shows confidence interval (CI). Vertical line represents no effect.
d. Overall estimate from the meta-analysis.
e. Pooled point estimate.

3.

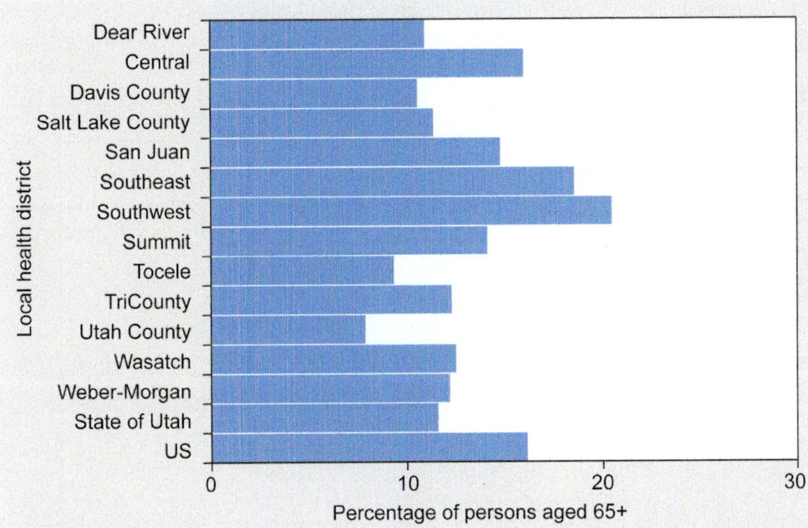

a. Identify the graph.
b. How do you identify the mode of this data?
c. What information is required to calculate mean from this data?
d. How is this graph different from histogram?

Ans.

a. Bar diagram.
b. The longest bar (southwest) represents the mode.
c. Population of each place would be required to calculate the mean.
d. Histogram has spaces in between the bars.

4.

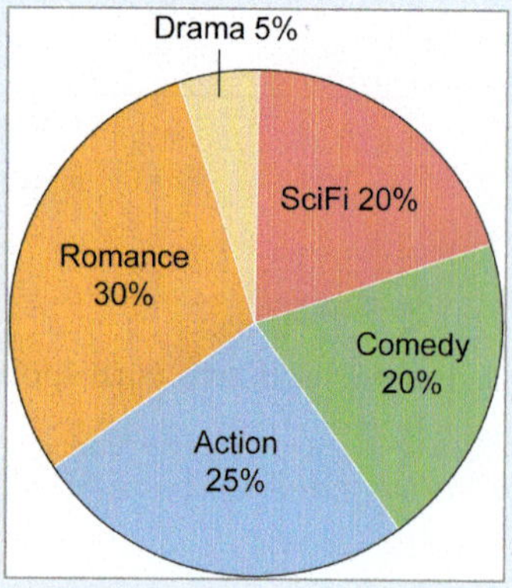

a. Identify the graph.
b. Which type of data display would you use it?
c. What do the segments in the graph represent?
d. What does the complete circle represent?

Ans.

a. Pie chart.
b. Qualitative data.
c. Segments represent the percentage of the whole.
d. A circle represents the 100% of variable of interest.

5.

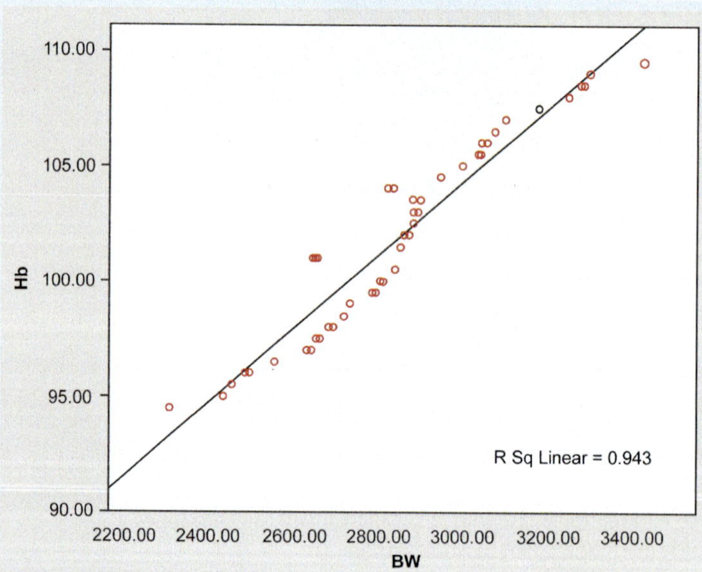

a. Identify the graph.
b. What is it used to represent?
c. What is positive and negative correlation?
d. What is line of best fit?

Ans.

a. Scatter plot.
b. Continuous numerical data between two groups.
c. It shows the relationship of one variable to another. When the "y" variable tends to increase or decrease as the "x" variable increases or decreases, we say there is a positive or negative correlation between the variables.
d. It refers to a line through a scatter plot of data points that best expresses the relationship between those points.

6.

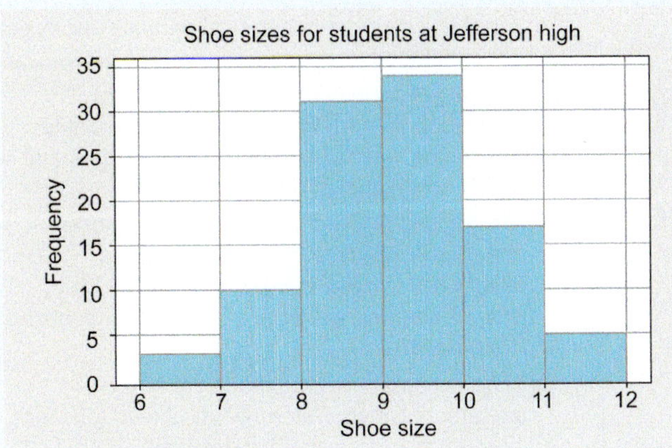

a. Identify the graph.
b. Why is it not a bar diagram?
c. What is the dependent and independent variable here?
d. Interpret the data displayed here.
e. What are the different shapes of this graphical display?
f. Name two uses of this display.
g. What parameter affects the shape of the histogram?

Ans.

a. Histogram.
b. Bar diagram has spaces between bars.
c. Shoe size is the independent variable. Dependent variable is the number or frequency of students with each shoe size.
d. Distribution is fairly symmetric with center of shoe size at 9.
e. Symmetric, right or left skewed deviation, bell shaped, and uniform.
f. Helps to identify patterns of display of data, helps comparison of two data sets, helps identify outliers, helps to identify whether the data set is unimodal or bimodal.
g. Bin width.

7. Match the trial with the objective of the study.

1. NANO trial 2. TOBY trial 3. BARNARDS study 4. NeoOBS study 5. DIAMOND trial 6. Baby-OSCAR	a. Determinants of outcomes after head cooling for neonatal encephalopathy b. Prospective multi-institutional randomized controlled trial to determine the safety of early antibiotic use in extremely low birth weight (ELBW) infants c. Neonatal sepsis and mortality in low-income and middle-income countries from a facility-based birth cohort: An international multisite prospective observational study d. Moderate hypothermia to treat perinatal asphyxial encephalopathy e. Patterns of antibiotic use, pathogens, and prediction of mortality in hospitalized neonates and young infants with sepsis: A global neonatal sepsis observational cohort study f. Efficacy and safety of short-course antibiotic therapy (72 hours) compared to standard duration (5–7 days) in preterm neonates with culture-negative early-onset sepsis: A randomized control trial g. Different approaches to moderate and late preterm nutrition: Determinants of feed tolerance, body composition and development h. Outcome after selective early treatment for closure of patent ductus arteriosus in preterm babies-a statistical analysis plan for short-term outcomes

Ans. 1-b, 2-d, 3-c, 4-e, 5-f, 6-g

8. Match the statistical test with its utility.

Statistical test	*Clinical application*
1. Fishers exact test 2. Chi-square test 3. Students t test 4. Mann–Whitney U test 5. Pearson correlation test	a. Investigates whether the expected values for two groups are the same, assuming that the data are normally distributed b. Suitable for binary data in unpaired samples c. Compare more than two groups or more than two categories of the outcome variable d. Tests whether two continuous normally distributed variables exhibit linear correlation e. Test for ordinal or continuous data f. Test preconditions as for the unpaired t-test, for comparison of more than two groups

Ans. 1-b, 2-c, 3-a, 4-e, 5-d

9. Match the study design with its clinical application.

Study design	*Clinical application*
1. Cross sectional study 2. Case series 3. Case control studies 4. Cohort study 5. Randomized control trial	a. To define the natural history of disease b. To assess the prevalence of a condition c. To assess the incidence of a disease or some other outcome d. To help determine if an exposure is associated with an outcome e. To study dose-response relationship between the cause and effect f. Comparison of two or more treatment strategies

Ans. 1-b, 2-a, 3-d, 4-c, 5-f

10. Match the existing relation between two different variables.

Measure of association	*Interpretation*
1. Attributable risk 2. Disease odds ratio 3. Relative risk 4. NNT	a. Shows what the chances are of getting this or that result. b. Shows how increased or decreased the risk of a given event is based on the event group. c. The number of times the risk of having an event is increased o reduced based on exposure. d. To assess the estimate of a measure. e. Estimated using the inverse of the absolute difference of incidences.

Ans. 1-b, 2-a, 3-c, 4-e

11.

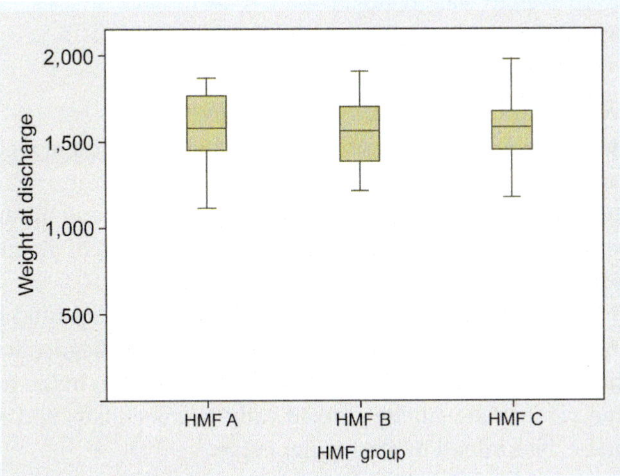

a. Identify.
b. What data display is it used for?
c. What data is displayed?
d. What does the central line in the box indicate?

Ans.

a. Box and whisker plot.
b. *Continuous numerical data:* ≥2 groups (Skewed data).
c. It is a 5 number summary of a set of data.
d. Median.

12.

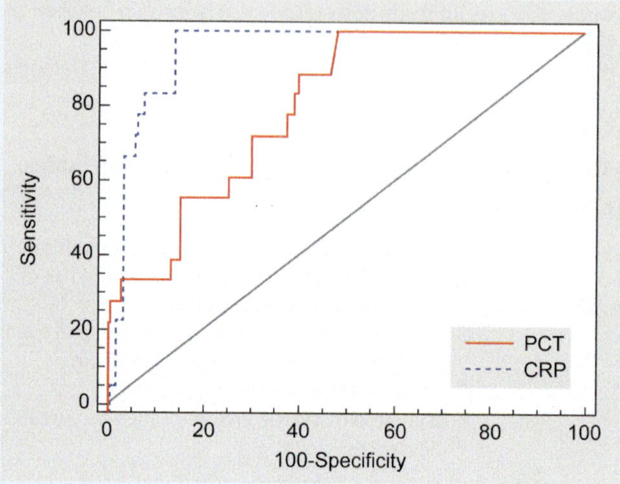

a. Identify.
b. What is it used for?
c. How do you interpret area under curve?
d. Name two uses.

Ans.

a. Receiver operating characteristic (ROC) curve
b. It is a graphical plot for selecting optimal cutoff for a test and comparing accuracy of diagnostic tests.
c. The area under the curve for the good test is close to 1 and the area under the curve for the poor test is close to 0.5 (50% chance of diagnosing the disease).
d. Shows all possible cutoff points and we can select optimal cutoff for identifying diseased and nondiseased, two or more diagnostic tests can be visually compared simultaneously in one figure, helps to identify required value of sensitivity at fixed value of specificity, and validity of test can be determined by area under curve.

13. Match the study with the standard reporting guidelines.

Study	*Reporting Guideline*
1. Randomized control trial 2. Cohort study 3. Diagnostic study test 4. Meta-analysis of RCT 5. Meta-analysis of observational studies	a. QUADAS b. CONSORT c. STROBE d. STARD e. PRISMA f. MOOSE g. QUROM

Ans. 1-b, 2-c, 3-d, 4-e, 5-f

14. You aim to test utility of polymerase chain reaction (PCR) for rapid diagnosis of sepsis. You compare PCR with blood culture as gold standard. Your results are as follows:

	Blood culture +ve (n)	*Blood culture –ve (n)*
PCR test +ve	9	4
PCR test –ve	0	87

Calculate sensitivity, specificity, positive predictive value, and negative predictive value for your results.

Ans.

	Blood culture +ve (n)	*Blood culture –ve (n)*
PCR test +ve	9 (a) True positive	4 (b) False positive
PCR test –ve	0 (c) False negative	87 (d) True negative

Sensitivity = a/a + c = 9/9 = 100%
Specificity= d/b + d =87/91 = 0.956 = 95.6%
Positive predictive value = a/a + b = 9/13 = 0.692 = 69.2%
Negative predictive value = d/c + d = 87/87 = 1 = 100%

CHAPTER

4.9

Genetics

1.

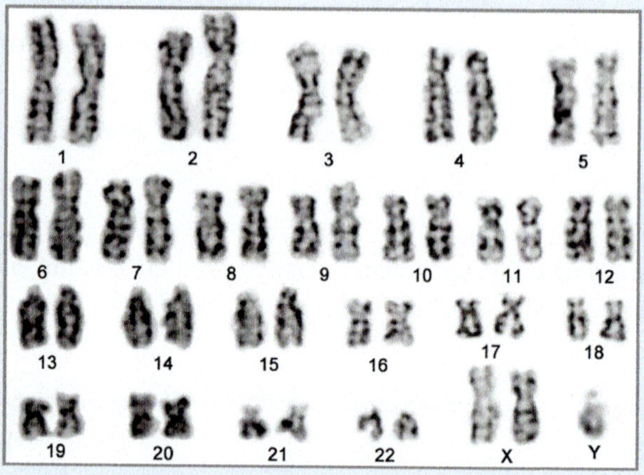

a. Identify the test and interpret the result.
b. Name two nonblood specimens on which this test is performed.
c. Name the most common sex chromosome abnormality in males.
d. Name a monosomy.
e. What is the turnaround time with this test?
f. Name four indications for this test.
g. Name two limitations.

Ans.

a. Karyotype, 46,XX.
b. Bone marrow aspirate, amniotic fluid, and chorionic villus sampling from placenta
c. Klinefelter syndrome, 46,XXY.
d. Turner syndrome, 46,XO.
e. 1–2 weeks.
f. Dysmorphic syndrome, disorder of sexual differentiation, short stature girl, and recurrent pregnancy losses.
g. Needs viable tissue, detects only major structural anomalies (5 Mb length resolution), cannot detect subtle deletions, duplications or rearrangements, labor intensive, and skill dependent.

2.

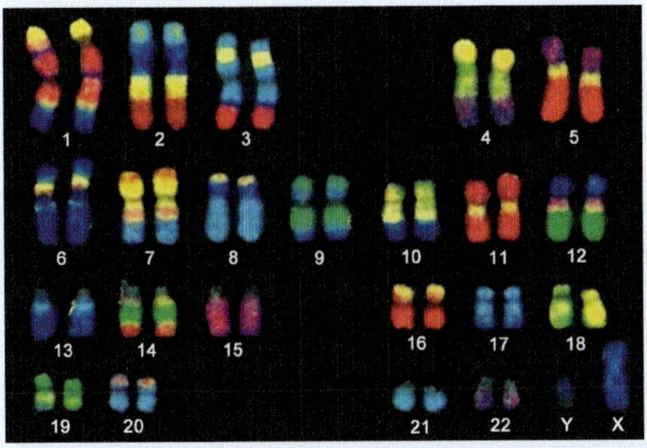

a. Identify the test.
b. What does it detect?
c. Name two indications.
d. What is the turnaround time with this test?
e. Name two limitations.
f. What specimen is required for testing?

Source: Carr SM. (2008). Fluorescent In-Situ Hybridization (FISH) identification of Human Chromosomes—"Chromosome Painting". [online] Available from https://www.mun.ca/biology/scarr/FISH_chromosome_painting.html. [Last accessed November, 2024].

Ans.

a. Fluorescence in situ hybridization (FISH).
b. It detects balanced and unbalanced rearrangements, and numerical changes of autosomes and sex chromosomes.
c. Specific clinical syndromes, suspected aneuploidies of chromosomes X/Y/13/18/21 prenatally/postnatally, syndromes caused due to specific microdeletions/duplication, viz., DiGeorge syndrome and William syndrome.
d. 2–4 days.
e. Smaller mutations cannot be identified (<2 Mb length), cannot be used in unknown genetic syndromes, probes not available for all chromosomal regions.
f. Heparinized blood.

3.

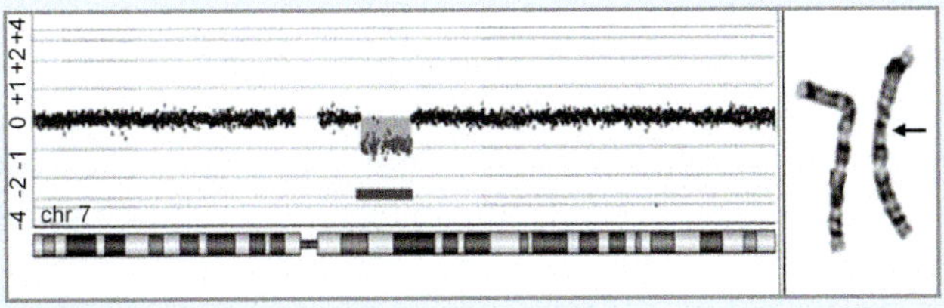

a. Identify the test.
b. Name four indications.
c. Name two limitations.
d. Name two advantages.
e. How does it differ from karyotype?
f. What is the turnaround time?

Ans.

a. Chromosomal microarray.
b. Significant dysmorphic features, unexplained developmental delay/ intellectual disability, autism spectrum disorders or nonsyndromic multiple congenital anomalies, and multiple miscarriages.
c. Cannot detect truly balanced rearrangements and low-level mosaicism.
d. Can detect deletions and duplications (25–50 kb), can detect single and contiguous gene syndromes, helpful for unknown or new clinical syndromes.
e. Does not require cell cultures or dividing cells.
f. 10 days.

4.

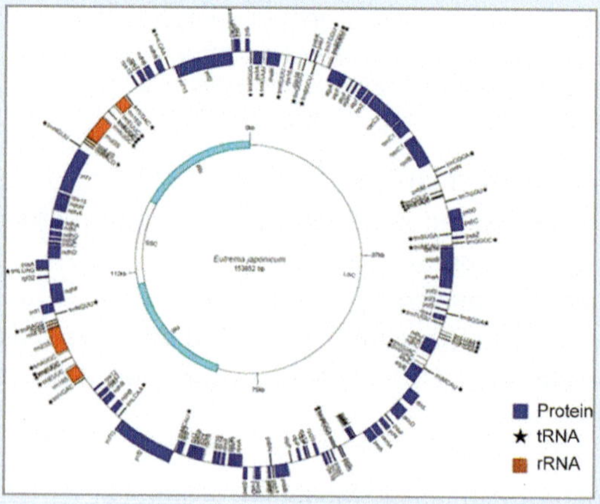

a. Identify the test.
b. What does it detect?
c. Name two limitations.
d. What does it not detect?
e. What is the standard turnaround time?

Ans.

a. Whole genome sequencing.
b. It detects coding and noncoding sequences, circulating DNA, copy number variation (CNV), and genomic structural rearrangements (translocations, etc.).
c. Increased risk of incidental findings (IFs) and variants of uncertain significance (VUS).
d. Deletions and duplications, intronic errors, trinucleotide errors, mosaicism, methylation errors, and mitochondrial DNA mutation.
e. 10–12 weeks.

5. Match the column.

1. Chromosomal abnormality	a. Beckwith–Wiedemann syndrome
2. Genomic disorder	b. Osteogenesis imperfecta
3. Single gene disorder	c. DiGeorge syndrome
4. Methylation defect	d. Cri-du-chat syndrome

Ans. 1-d, 2-c, 3-b, 4-a

6. Match the clinical features with the genetic syndrome.

1. Turners syndrome	a. Neonatal hypotonia, feeding difficulties
2. Prader–Willi syndrome	b. Cystic hygroma, webbed neck, CoA, renal abnormalities
3. Cornelia de Lange syndrome	c. Distinctive facies, cholestatic jaundice, bile duct paucity on liver biopsy, butterfly vertebrae, posterior embryotoxon, TOF
4. Alagille syndrome	d. Growth retardation, hirsutism, synophrys, highly arched eyebrows, upper limb reduction defects
5. Noonan syndrome	e. Hydrops, dysmorphic features, pulmonary valve stenosis, HCM, cryptorchidism

Ans. 1-b, 2-a, 3-d, 4-c, 5-e

7.

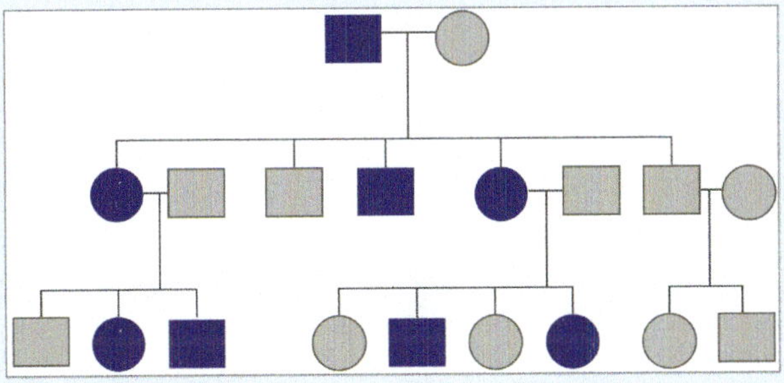

a. Identify the mode of inheritance.
b. What is the risk of transmission to the next generation?
c. Name two cardiac disorders with this mode of inheritance.
d. Name two bone disorders with this mode of inheritance.
e. Why is there no gender preference in inheritance?

Ans.

a. Autosomal dominant.
b. 50%.
c. Hypertrophic cardiomyopathy and heredity long QT syndrome.
d. Achondroplasia and osteogenesis imperfecta.
e. Disease gene is autosomal (i.e., not on a sex chromosome).

8.

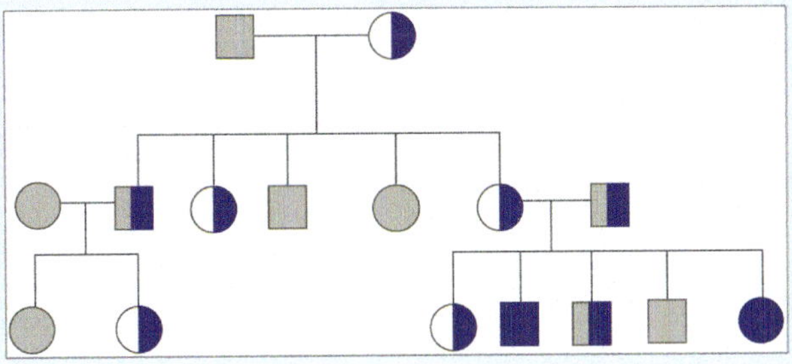

a. Identify the mode of inheritance.
b. What is the risk of transmission to the next-generation if both the parents are carriers?
c. What is the risk of transmission to the next-generation if one parent is a carrier and the other with disease?
d. What is the risk of transmission to the next-generation if one parent is a carrier?
e. Name two blood disorders with this mode of inheritance.

Ans.

a. Autosomal recessive.
b. 25% chance of disease, 25% chance of being normal, and 50% chance of being a carrier.
c. 50% chance of disease.
d. 50% chance of carrier.
e. Sickle cell disease and thalassemia.

9.

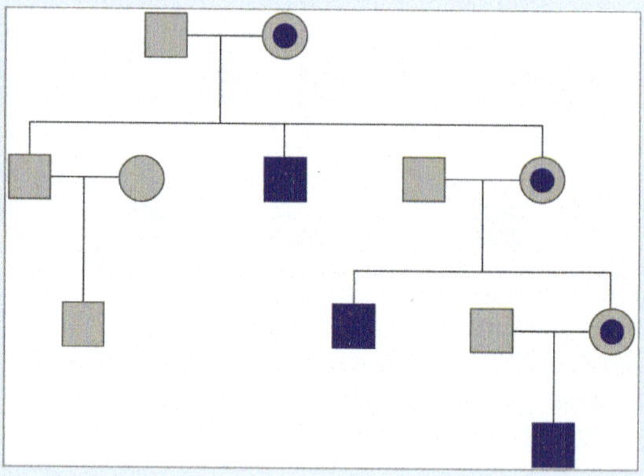

a. Identify the mode of inheritance.
b. What is the risk of male to male transmission?
c. What is the risk to son and daughter of a carrier mother?
d. What is the risk to daughters from affected father?
e. Name two blood disorders with this mode of inheritance.

Ans.

a. X-linked inheritance.
b. Not possible.
c. 50% risk of affection in boys, 50% risk of being carrier in girls.
d. All the daughters will be carriers.
e. Factor VIII deficiency, factor IX deficiency, and glucose-6-phosphate dehydrogenase (G6PD) deficiency.

10.

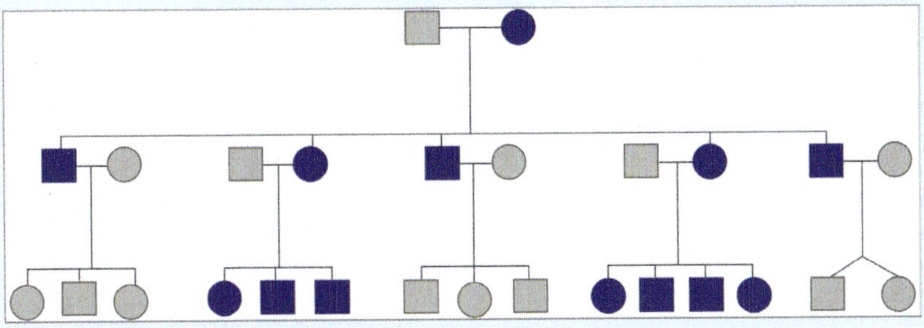

a. Identify the mode of inheritance.
b. Why affected males do not transmit the disease?
c. Name two body parts most commonly affected.
d. What is the most common time of presentation?

Ans.

a. Only affected females transmit the disease—mitochondrial inheritance.
b. As sperm do not contribute mitochondria to the zygote, affected males do not transmit the disease.
c. Neurons and muscles.
d. Puberty.

CHAPTER 4.10

Special Investigations

1. This male term newborn presents with abdominal distension and oliguria on the second day after birth.

a. What test is shown here and what are the findings?

b. What is the classical prenatal scan finding for this case?

c. When and what intervention is done in this newborn?

d. What are the long-term complications of this condition?

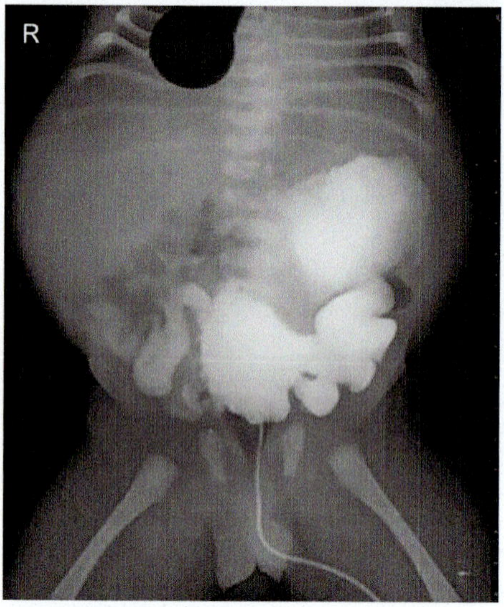

Ans.

a. Micturating cystourethrogram is done here and it is showing trabeculated bladder and dilated and tortuous urethra and hydronephrosis.

b. Keyhole appearance of the bladder outlet.

c. If the renal functions are normal, then the newborn will be subjected to fulguration of the posterior urethral valve. If not a vesicostomy is done initially till renal functions improve.

d. Renal failure, recurrent urinary tract infection (UTI), and bladder dysfunction.

2. **This newborn presents 4 weeks after a tracheoesophageal fistula (TEF) surgery with complains of feed intolerance, vomiting, and poor weight gain:**

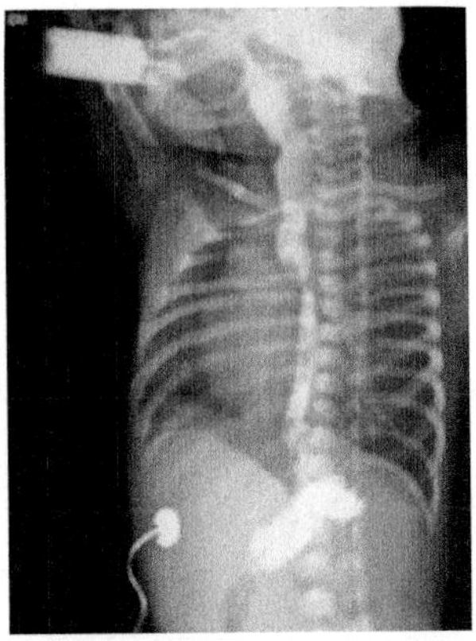

a. **What is the test performed and what are the findings?**
b. **What are the complications of TEF surgery?**
c. **What is the treatment for this condition?**
d. **What is the primary surgery for TEF if the gap between esophageal stump and lower esophagus is >2 cm?**

Ans.

a. Upper gastrointestinal (GI) contrast study. There is a stricture in the midesophagus.
b. Stricture, gastroesophageal reflux disease (GERD), chylothorax, and anastomosis leaks.
c. Balloon dilation of the stricture.
d. Gastrostomy and esophageal ostia in the neck.

3. **This newborn presents with abdominal distension and bilious aspirates:**

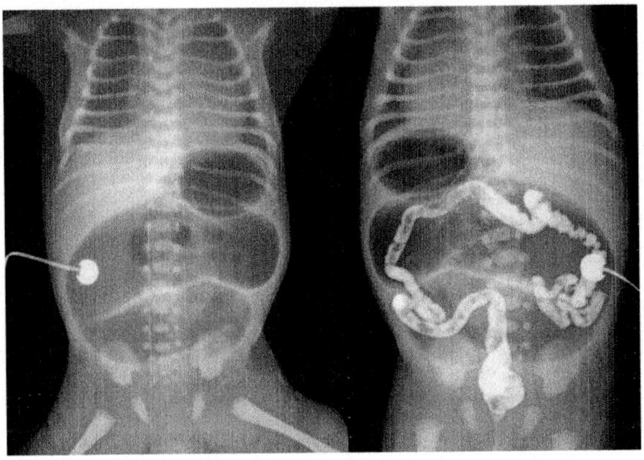

a. What the tests and what are the findings?
b. What is diagnosis?
c. What is the most important medical management in jejunal atresia?
d. What are the findings of Hirschsprung on lower GI contrast?

Ans.

a. Abdominal X-ray and lower GI contrast. Dilated bowel loops, triple bubble sign. Colon and long intestine of low caliber
b. Intestinal atresia or jejunal atresia
c. Total parenteral nutrition
d. Rectosigmoid ratio <1. Reduced caliber of rectum, transition zone, and proximal dilatation of Sigmoid and colon

4.

a. What is this spinal defect and its association shown?
b. What are the prognostic features of this defect?
c. How to prevent this defect in subsequent pregnancy?
d. What is the primary prevention for this condition?

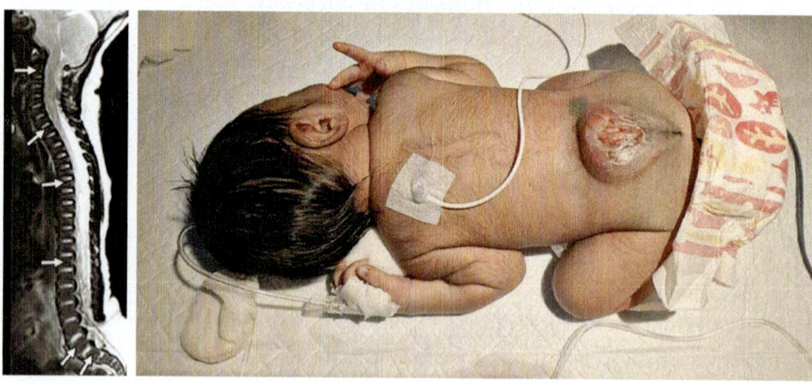

Ans.

a. Open spinal tube defect. Myelomeningocele. Arnold Chiari malformation type II is shown here with tonsillar herniation.
b. Higher the defect, open defects, gestation, and associated defects are the major prognostic factors of this defect.
c. 4 mg once daily folate 1 month prior to 3 months of pregnancy
d. 0.5 mg once daily to all pregnant mothers in the first 3 months of pregnancy

5.

a. What is the image shown here? What are the findings in this image?
b. What all can be prognosticated using this imaging modality?
c. Name four neonatal morbidities and their classical findings on this imaging.

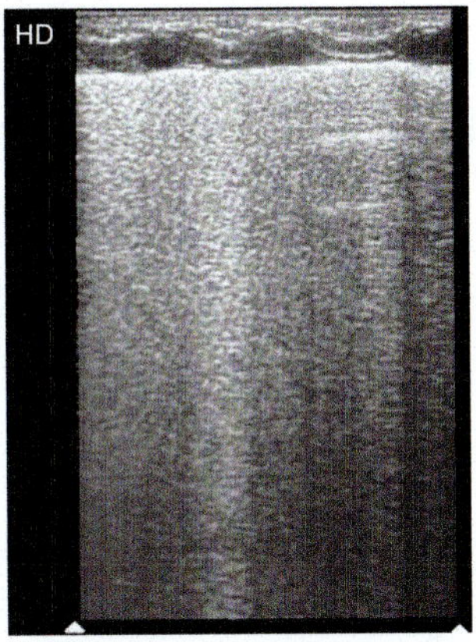

Ans.

a. This image of lung ultrasound showing double lung point. Half of the image is showing B lines and other half showing A lines.
b. Need for surfactant and ventilation can be predicted using lung ultrasound scoring.
c. The five morbidities with their classical findings are:
    1. *Respiratory distress syndrome (RDS):* Thickened pleura, coalescent or compact B lines, and subpleural breaks
    2. *Transient tachypnea of the newborn (TTNB):* Double lung point, alveolar interstitial pattern
    3. *Pneumothorax:* Absence of lung sliding and stratosphere sign
    4. *Pleural effusion:* Collection of subpleural space
    5. *Pneumonia:* Shred sign

6. What are these two growth charts and what information is presented here?

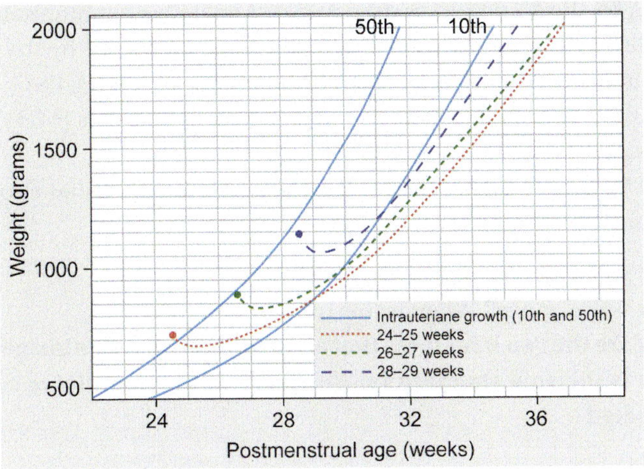

Ans.

- Two growth charts are shown here, an intrauterine growth chart with 10th and 50%th centile and a postnatal growth chart of babies of extreme preterm infants.
- All extreme preterm are extrauterine growth restricted when they reach the term corrected age or 36 week of postmenstrual age (PMA).

7.

a. What are these curves used for?

b. What does A, B and C lines represent?

c. What are the interventions for each of the categories?

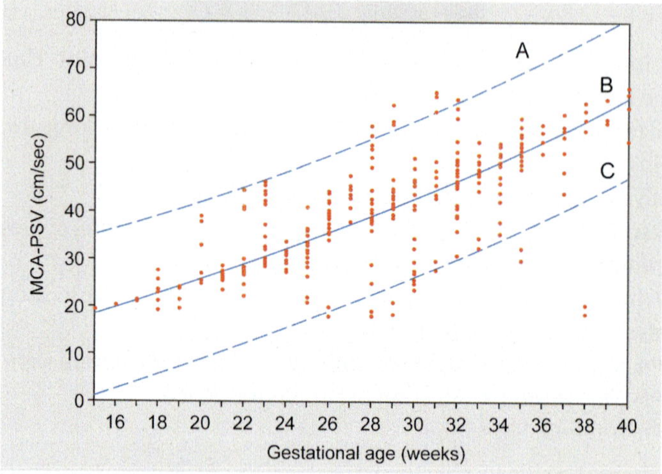

Ans.

a. These are the Marie curves used to assess fetal Rh isoimmunization.

b. The lines represent the severity of anemia as reflected by the increase in middle cerebral artery peak systolic velocity (MCA-PSV) velocity. MCA-PSV velocity is represented by multiple of medians (MoM) for that gestation.

c. If the MoM is >1.5, the fetal needs fetal blood sampling and also in utero transfusion.

8.

a. What is the image? When is this used?

b. What are the two structures that are highlighted in this image?

c. What is the gold standard for diagnosis of the underlying condition evaluated?

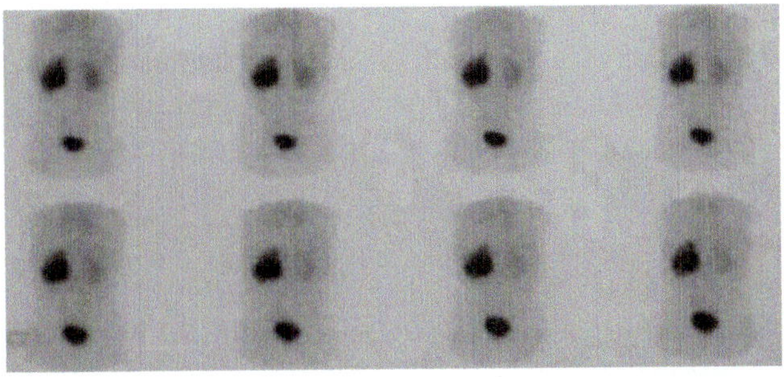

Ans.

a. The image is that of hepatobiliary iminodiacetic acid (HIDA) scan. It is used to see the dye is excreted from liver to intestines. Absence of dye in the intestine is a feature of extrahepatic biliary atresia.
b. Liver and urinary bladder are highlighted in the image.
c. The gold standard is peroperative cholangiogram and biopsy.

9.

a. What is image?
b. When is this image used?
c. What is the gold standard in the diagnosis of the underlying disease evaluated?

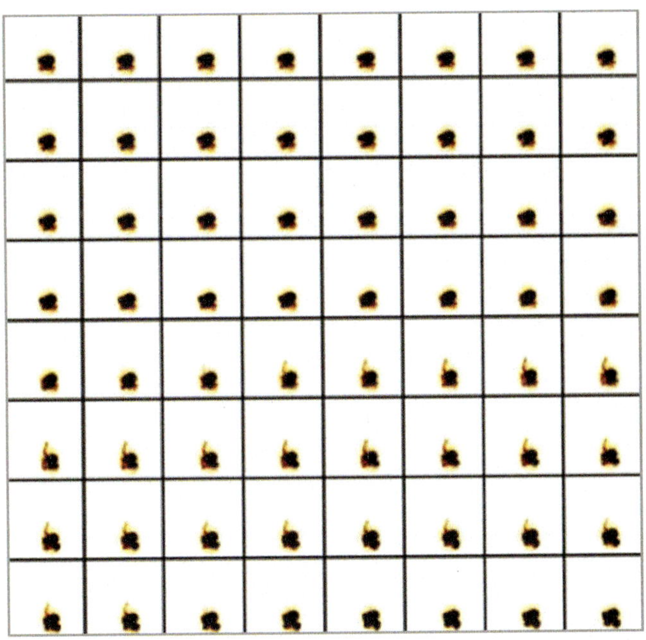

Ans.

a. This image is that of nuclear milk scan for evaluation of GERD.
b. This image is useful to evaluate the presence and severity of GERD.
c. 24-hour intraesophageal pH monitoring is the gold standard for diagnosis of GERD.

10.

a. What is this image?
b. What isotopes are commonly used for this purpose?
c. When is this used?
d. What is the interpretation of this graph and image?

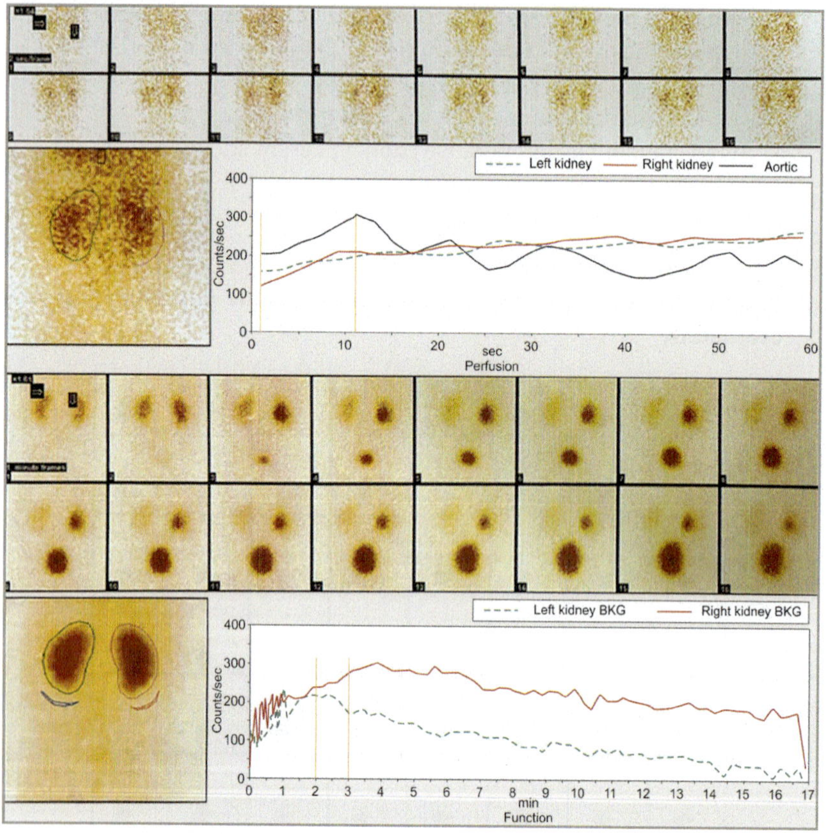

Ans.

a. This is radioisotope renogram. It measures the perfusion, filtration, and drainage functions of kidneys.
b. MAG3 and DPTA are the common isotopes used. MAG3 is used if renogram is required in the first 6 weeks after birth and DTPA if needed later.

c. Normally renogram is used if hydronephrosis is diagnosed either prenatal or immediate postnatal but it is usually done after 6 weeks after birth. In case of severe hydronephrosis, the test may be done immediately but using MAG3.

d. Both the kidneys are well perfused. Drainage of tracer is smooth in the left kidney but is delayed in right kidney. Drainage is complete in right kidney at the end of 17 minutes.

   If the differential renal function is <40% in one of the kidneys and if there is obstructive pattern a surgical intervention is needed.

5

SECTION

Neonatal Resuscitation

CHAPTER 5.1

Neonatal Resuscitation

SETTING

You are a resident on call in delivery room. A case scenario will be given. Proceed with steps of resuscitation.

TASK

- Demonstrate the step of resuscitation on manikin.
- You may talk as you perform the step.
- You may take help of an attendant during the procedure.
- You may ask for any information as you proceed.

DURATION

10 minutes

EVALUATION

Correct/missed/incorrect

CASE 1

A term newborn is just born and is crying. There are no risk factors in the mother. How do you assess and manage at birth?

Demonstrate routine care	
Tick here	*Step*
	• Assess if breathing is well (Yes)
	• Postpones cord clamping for at least 1 minute
	• Keeps baby on mother's abdomen. Covers the baby with a dry, clean cloth
	• Ensures clear airway, suctions if visible secretions
	• Dries the baby, cuts the cord
	• Ensures the baby is dry by removing wet linen
	• Gives to mother for early skin to skin contact
	• Asks the mother to initiate breastfeeding
	• Indicates no separation of mother and baby, need for frequent monitoring of temperature, breathing, and activity

CASE 2

A newborn is apneic after initial steps of resuscitation. You may ask for relevant details as you proceed to manage this case.

Demonstrate positive pressure ventilation	
Tick here	*Step*
	• Indicates need for positive pressure ventilation (PPV)
	• Calls for help; requests for pulse oximeter
	• Positions mask correctly
	• Delivers adequate pressure to get chest rise
	• Ventilates at appropriate rate (breathe-two-three to achieve 40–60/min)
	• Requests heart rate (HR) response after providing up to 15 test breaths
HR 40 beats/min, no breath sounds heard	
	Takes corrective steps for ventilation: • Reapplies mask • Repositions baby head Assess for chest rise and breath sounds (no chest rise and breath sounds) • Suctions mouth • Ventilates with mouth open Assess for chest rise and breath sounds (no chest rise and breath sounds) • Increases bag pressure (there is chest rise)
	Administers effective PPV for 30 seconds
	Asks for HR (HR is 120 beats/min and baby is breathing well)
	Gradually discontinues PPV after confirming spontaneous breathing
	Indicates need for observational care for the baby

CASE 3

A term, newborn is just born. There is meconium-stained amniotic fluid (MSAF). How do you manage?

Meconium-stained liquor delivery	
Tick here	*Step*
	Asks for respiration, heart rate, and tone (baby is not breathing and limp)
	Identifies baby needs resuscitation
	Cuts the cord and shifts baby under warmer
	Ensures clear airway, suctions if visible secretions
	Dries the baby from head to trunk, abdomen, back, and limbs
	Removes wet linen and repositions the baby to sniffing position
	Requests breathing and heart rate *(Not breathing)*

Contd...

Contd...

Tick here	*Step*
	• Calls for help; requests for pulse oximeter
	• Positions mask correctly
	• Delivers adequate pressure to get chest rise
	• Ventilates at appropriate rate (Breathe-two-three to achieve 40–60/min)
	• Requests HR response after providing up to 15 test breaths *(HR is 70 beats/min)*
	Takes corrective steps for ventilation: • Reapplies mask • *Repositions baby head:* Assess for chest rise and breath sounds (no chest rise and breath sounds) • Suctions mouth. Intubates and under vision performs tracheal suction applying suction pressure during tube withdrawal. Requests attendant to monitor HR • *Ventilates with mouth open:* Assess for chest rise and breath sounds (no chest rise and breath sounds) • Increases bag pressure (there is chest rise)
	Administers effective PPV for 30 seconds
	Asks for HR (HR is 120 beats/min and baby is breathing well)
	Gradually discontinues PPV after confirming spontaneous breathing
	Indicates need for observational care for the baby

STATION 1

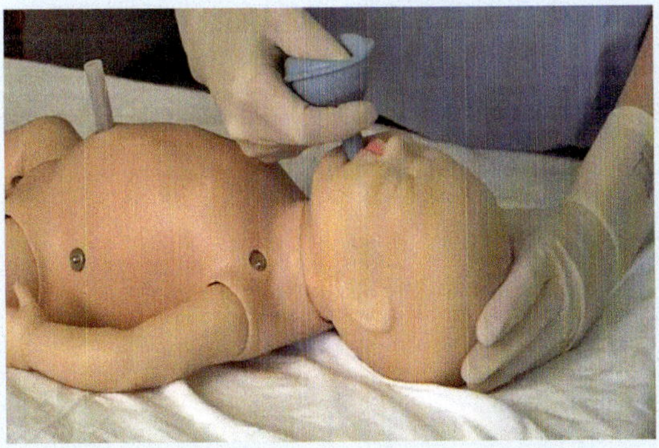

a. Identify two errors in this step.
b. Name two indications for this step.
c. Name two complications for this step.
d. What should be the pressure cut off?

Ans.

a. Using suction bulb, not turning the head to one side
b. Visible secretions, prior to starting PPV, during ventilation corrective measures
c. Bradycardia, hypoxia, soft tissue injury, and apnea
d. 100 mm Hg

STATION 2

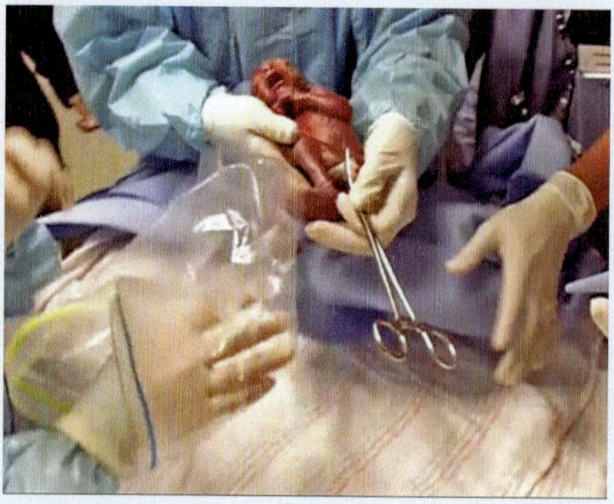

a. Identify the step.
b. Below what gestation do you offer this step.
c. Which step of resuscitation do you skip while doing this?
d. Name two other measures you take along with this step for thermal care.

Ans.

a. Receiving preterm in food grade plastic
b. <32 weeks
c. You skip the initial steps.
d. Cover the head with cap, ensure warmer is on skin mode at 36°C, use thermal mattress, and use warm humidified gases.

STATION 3

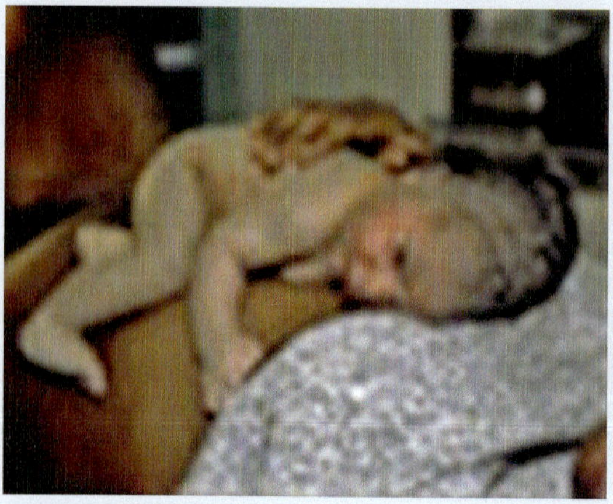

a. Identify the step in delivery room.
b. Above what gestation do you offer this step.
c. When do you skip this step?
d. Name two benefits to the mother.

Ans.

a. Skin-to-skin contact
b. Above 30 weeks of gestation
c. If the baby needs resuscitation
d. Early breastfeeding, boosts bonding

STATION 4

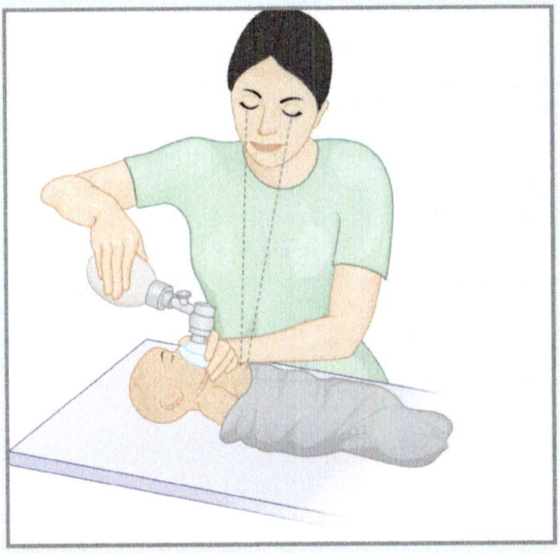

a. Name the four components of first golden minute.
b. When do you first check the heart rate with PPV?
c. Name two contraindications for PPV.
d. What do you check first to define effectiveness of PPV?

Ans.

a. Assess need for resuscitation at birth, perform initial steps, reassess breathing and heart rate, and initiate PPV not later than 1 minute.
b. 15 seconds
c. Suspected congenital diaphragmatic hernia, pneumothorax
d. Rise in heart rate

STATION 5

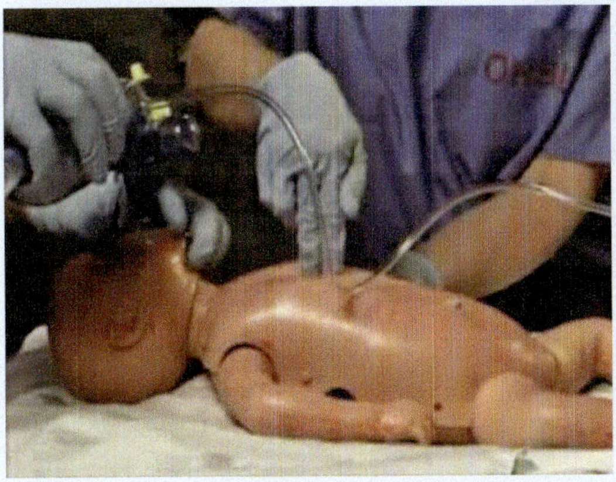

a. Identify two errors in this step.
b. Name two mandatory steps with this.
c. What is the preferred method to check HR?
d. Below what HR do you perform this step.

Ans.

a. Using two finger technique, using bag, and mask ventilation
b. Performing intubation, using 100% oxygen
c. Cardiac monitor
d. HR <60 beats/min

STATION 6

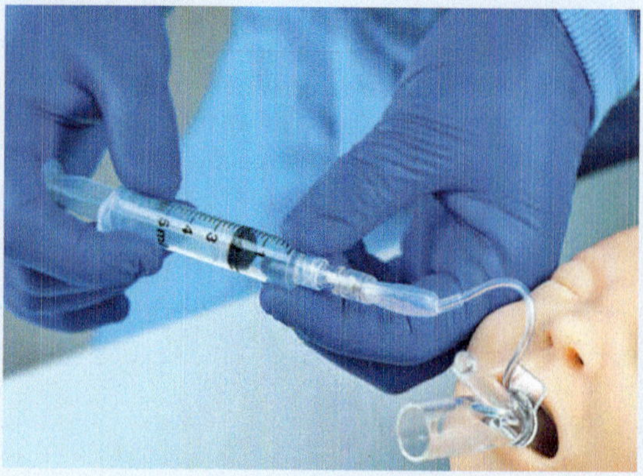

a. Identify the equipment.
b. Name two indications.
c. Name four limitations.
d. Name two disadvantages.

Ans.

a. Laryngeal mask airway
b. Cannot intubate, cannot ventilate, facial anomalies
c. Not for <35 weeks, not for <2 kg, not for meconium-stained liquor suction, and not for medication administration
d. Risk of gastric insufflation and aspiration, cannot deliver >25 cm H_2O pressure leading to inadequate alveolar ventilation, needs practice.

STATION 7

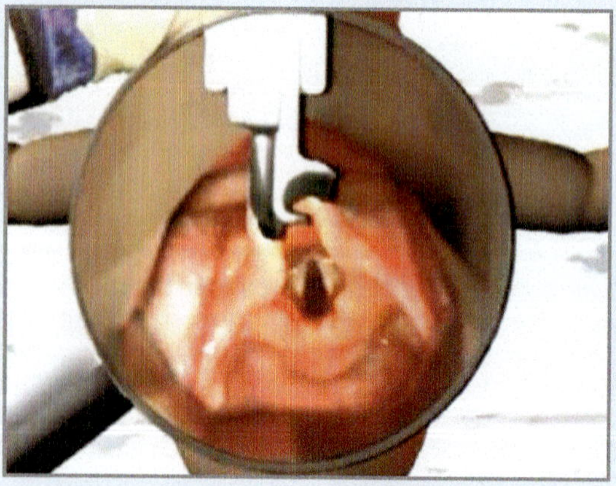

a. Within what time frame should you perform this step?
b. What is the fastest way to decide depth of insertion of endotracheal (ET) tube?
c. Which is the most reliable way to decide ET tube size and depth?
d. Is cricoid pressure during procedure recommended?

Ans.

a. Within 30 seconds
b. Nasotragal length plus 1 cm
c. Based on weight and gestation
d. No

STATION 8

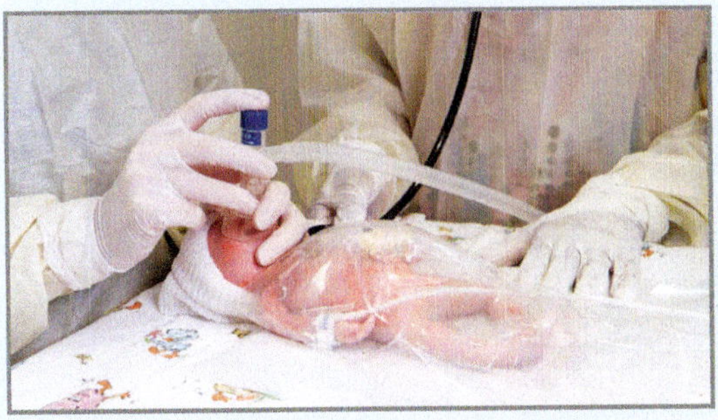

a. Name two advantages of this over bag and mask ventilation.
b. Name four disadvantages.
c. What is the preferred method to check HR with this step?

Ans.

a. Delivers consistent pressures independent of operator experience, *delivers consistent and controlled PEEP, can deliver desired oxygen concentration.*
b. Needs compressed gas, blender, unknown tidal volume, training, difficult to change pressures during ventilation, and positive end-expiratory pressure (PEEP) changes with change in flow rate, costly.
c. Pulse oximeter

STATION 9

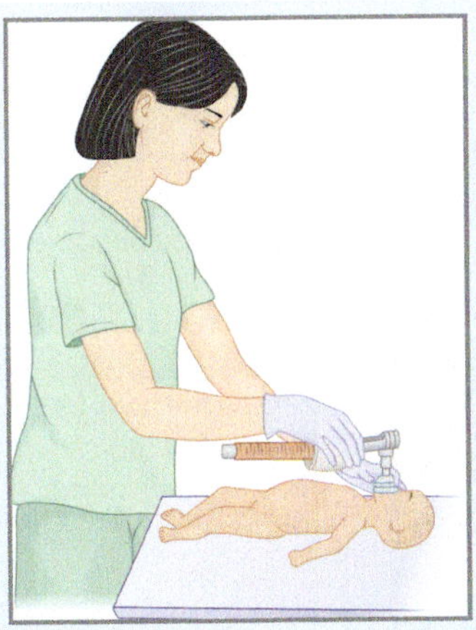

a. Identify the error in this step.
b. Name four potential complications of this step.
c. What do you assess if there is no rise in heart rate with this step?
d. Below what heart rate would you initiate this step?

Ans.

a. Standing at foot end of the baby
b. Ineffective ventilation due to leak, over or under ventilation, pulmonary air leak, chronic lung disease, gaseous distention interfering ventilation, difficult to perform over prolonged period, and risk of aspiration
c. Chest movement
d. HR below 100 beats/min

STATION 10

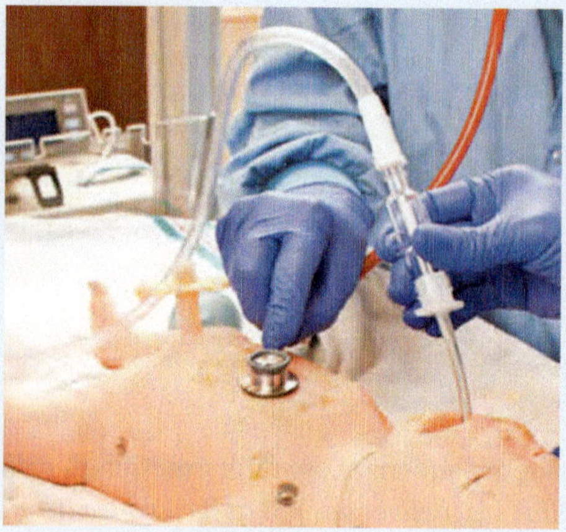

a. Identify the equipment.
b. What do you monitor during this step?
c. When do you use it?
d. How many times do you repeat this step?

Ans.

a. Meconium aspirator
b. Heart rate
c. In meconium-stained liquor, baby depressed at birth after initial steps and during ventilation corrective measure
d. Till meconium is clear provided HR is being maintained.

STATION 11

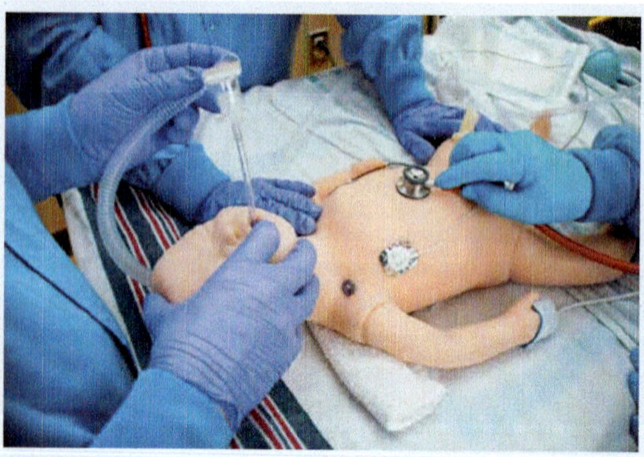

a. Identify two errors in this step.
b. How do you measure the distance for insertion of orogastric tube?
c. What is the preferred pulse oximeter technology in delivery room?

Ans.

a. Long ET tube, checking air entry over abdomen
b. From bridge of nose to ear lobe, point midway between xiphoid and umbilicus
c. Signal extraction technology

STATION 12

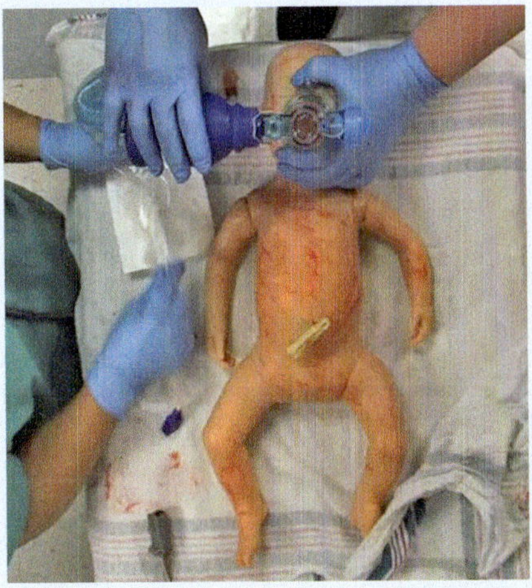

1. What should be oxygen concentration for:
   a. PPV in 36 weeks
   b. TPR in 28 weeks
   c. During chest compression
   d. Bag and mask ventilation with 10L of oxygen flow without reservoir
2. What interquartile range is used for target oxygen saturation during first 10 minutes?

Ans.

1. (a) 21 %; (b) 21–30%; (c)100%; (d) 40%
2. 25–75%

STATION 13

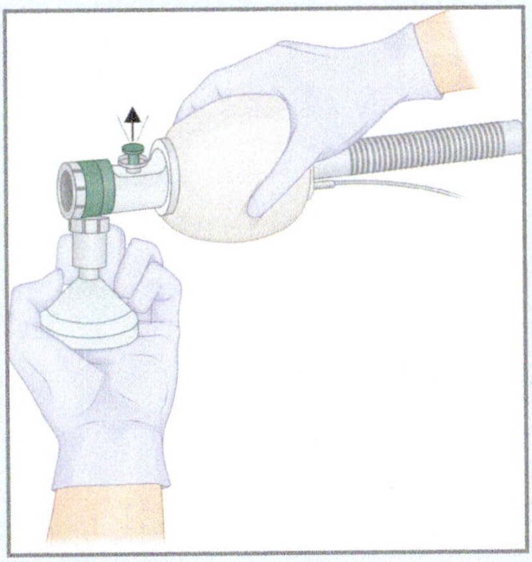

a. Name four features to suggest functional self-inflating bag.
b. What is the preferred method to sterilize this equipment?
c. How much should the flow of oxygen set for its use?

Ans.

a. Feels pressure on palm, pop off valve moves up and down, hissing sound, quick refill of bag, and movement on pressure gauge
b. Gas sterilization
c. 10 L/min

SECTION 6

Clinical Skill

CHAPTER 6.1

Procedure

TASK: DEMONSTRATE THE PROCEDURE

1. USING PULSE OXIMETER FOR NEWBORN SCREENING

Steps	*Tick here*
• Perform hand hygiene • Confirm patient identity and age (>24 hours)	
Identify appropriate site and probe.	
Place pulse oximeter probe on right upper palm.	
Switch on the pulse oximeter.	
Note the oxygen saturation reading.	
Repeat procedure on either of the foot and note reading.	
Interpret reading and note the difference between upper and lower limb.	
Document reading (the infant should be stable, waveform should be uniform, and heart rate by stethoscope should correlate with that on the pulse oximeter)	
• Identify *pass* if the saturation in both the limbs is >95% and a difference of 3% or less. • Identify *fail* if the saturation in right hand or foot is <90%. • Identify *retest* in 1 hour if the saturation in right hand or foot is 90–94% OR there is a difference of 4% or more between the right hand and foot.	

2. USING NONINVASIVE BLOOD PRESSURE MONITOR

Steps	*Tick here*
• Perform hand hygiene. • Confirm patient identity, gestation, and postnatal age. • Ensure infant is quiet or asleep.	
Identify appropriate site and cuff (the cuff bladder should measure two-thirds the length of the extremity and 0.50 of the arm circumference).	
Place blood pressure (BP) cuff on the upper arm with the cuff bladder width approximately 50% of the midarm circumference and length covering nearly 80% of arm circumference. Line up the cuff marker over the brachial artery.	

Contd...

Contd...

Steps	*Tick here*
Switch on the monitor. Wait for the infant to be calm. Note the systolic, diastolic, and mean BP reading [mean arterial pressure (MAP) is the most reliable reading]	
Take at least three BP readings.	
Interpret reading and note the difference between upper and lower limb.	
Document reading.	
Remove the cuff.	

3. USING THE DIGITAL THERMOMETER

Steps	*Tick here*
• Perform hand hygiene. • Confirm patient identity.	
• Ensure the armpit is dry.	
Place the tip of the thermometer parallel to the baby at the center of armpit. Close the armpit by moving the elbow to the chest. Ensure there is no clothing between the skin and the thermometer.	
Wait for the beep to note the display.	
Document reading.	
Remove the thermometer, clean and place it back in the case.	

4. GIVING INTRAMUSCULAR INJECTION FOR VITAMIN K

Steps	*Tick here*
• Perform hand hygiene. • Confirm patient identity. • Ensure all supplies are available.	
Use disposable, correct syringe (1 cc), correct 25-gauge, 25 mm needle.	
Draw the correct amount of the drug into the syringe.	
Identify site of administration—middle third of the thigh, in the outer anterolateral aspect, lateral to the midpoint of the thigh.	
Do not rub the site of administration with alcohol swab if the site is visibly clean.	
• Ensure the infant is comfortable in mother's lap or in lying down position • Ensure the infant does not move and the extremity is immobilized.	
Hold the needle perpendicular to the thigh.	
Administer the entire drug slowly into the muscle of the thigh.	
Remove needle. Check the site for bleeding and apply cotton.	
Ask the mother to breastfeed and report if there is any bleeding or redness at the site.	
Document administration.	
Discard syringe, needle appropriately.	

5. USING GLUCOMETER

Steps	*Tick here*
• Perform hand hygiene. • Confirm patient identity. • Ensure all supplies are available. • Wear clean gloves.	
Turn on the glucometer by inserting a test strip. Check the glucometer's screen, which alerts to add the blood sample to the strip.	
Wipe the side of the heel with alcohol swab and allow it to dry.	
Pierce the baby's side of heel using the lancing device (lancing pen).	
Place the blood sample on the test strip.	
Place cotton swab to stop bleeding at the puncture site.	
Note and document the displayed result.	
Turn off the glucometer, dispose test strip, and remove gloves.	
Wash hand.	

6. ENDOTRACHEAL INTUBATION

Steps	*Tick here*
• Perform hand hygiene. • Confirm patient identity. • Ensure all supplies are available. • Confirm patient is on monitor (pulse ox, multichannel) • Confirm assistant's presence • Identify size of endotracheal (ET) tube and depth of insertion. • Wear gloves.	
Choose appropriate-size ET tube, laryngoscope blade, and ensure bulb is functional.	
Stand at the head end of the patient. Place infant's head in neutral or sniffing position.	
Clear airway, if needed (suction).	
Hold laryngoscope in left hand and insert laryngoscope blade in right side of mouth, moving tongue to the left.	
Visualize epiglottis.	
Apply traction to the long axis of the laryngoscope handle to open the airway and visualize vocal cords.	
Insert the ET tube in the groove of the laryngoscope to proper length within 30 seconds.	
Provide bag to tube ventilation and look for chest rise. Ask assistant to check air entry.	
Secure ET tube in place.	
Ask for X-ray for confirmation.	
Remove gloves. Wash hand. Document procedure.	

7. LARYNGEAL MASK AIRWAY

Steps	*Tick here*
• Perform hand hygiene. • Confirm patient identity. • Ensure all supplies are available. • Confirm patient is on monitor (pulse oximeter, multichannel). • Confirm assistant's presence. • Identify size of laryngeal mask airway (LMA). • Wear gloves.	
Stand at the head end of patient. Place infant's head in neutral or sniffing position.	
Clear airway, if needed (suction).	
Hold LMA between three fingers of the right hand with the concavity up.	
Insert LMA into mouth and place it so that the curvature is the same as that of the pharynx, directing it posteriorly until resistance is felt.	
Inflate the cuff with the appropriate amount of air corresponding to the size of the tube, remove syringe.	
Provide bag to LMA, ventilation, and look for chest rise. Ask assistant to check air entry.	
Secures LMA in place.	
Remove gloves. Wash hand. Document procedure.	

8. PERIPHERAL INTRAVENOUS CANNULATION

Steps	*Tick here*
• Perform hand hygiene. • Confirm patient identity. • Ensure all supplies are available. • Wear gloves.	
Ensure the infant is comforted by massage, talk, and oral sucrose or breast milk. Ensure the infant does not move and the extremity is immobilized.	
Locate vein (by palpation) and cleanse the overlying skin with alcohol or povidone iodine. Wait for the disinfectant to dry.	
Hold vein in place and ask assistant to apply pressure on vein distal to the point of entry.	
Puncture the skin (in 15°–30°) with bevel of needle upward about ½ centimeter from the vein either from the side or from above.	
Note blood return, remove needle, and advance the catheter into the vein.	
Flush the catheter with 1 mL normal saline. Ensure patency and note no fullness, resistance, or blanching of skin.	
Attach infusion set to the needle.	
Ask the assistant to fix transparent dressing at the site of insertion.	
Remove gloves, dispose used supplies, and wash hands.	
Document procedure.	

9. MODIFIED ALLEN'S TEST

- Perform hand hygiene.
- Confirm patient identity.

Clench the patient's fist.

Apply pressure over the radial and ulnar artery to occlude both vessels.

Open the patient's hand. It should appear blanched. If not, it means you are not completely occluding the arteries.

Remove the pressure from the ulnar artery while maintaining pressure over the radial artery.

Normal color should appear within 5–15 seconds indicating adequate collateral circulation. If not, it suggests poor collateral circulation and one should avoid doing arterial blood gas (ABG) on this hand.

10. ARTERIAL PUNCTURE

- Perform hand hygiene.
- Confirm patient identity.
- Check adequacy of supplies.
- Perform modified Allen's test.

Hyperextend wrist and palpate radial artery with index and middle finger. Wear gloves.

Cleanse skin with povidone iodine and alcohol and allow to naturally dry.

Expel air from the heparinized syringe.

Use nondominant hand to repalpate radial artery with index and middle finger.

Insert the heparinized syringe with bevel up at 45° to the skin over the pulsations near the nondominant finger.

Allow flow of blood into the syringe and aspirate the sample.

Place cotton over the puncture site and withdraw needle from the skin. Apply firm pressure at the site over 5 minutes and ensure bleeding has stopped.

Secure the syringe with the needle cover and ask for immediate sample assessment. If the estimation is delayed place the syringe on dry ice and transport to laboratory.

Discard gloves. Wash hands.

Document procedure.

11. KANGAROO CARE

Introduce self, greet the mother, and inform purpose of visit.

Inform procedure of kangaroo mother care (KMC) to mother.

• Preparation: – Ensure privacy of mother. – Ensure room temperature is 26°–28°C and free of draught of air. – Ensure mother wears a front opening gown or shirt, which easily opens in front with bra removed. – Ensure mother is comfortable, clean, and has a toilet break beforehand. – Note chair is available and pillow for support. – Ensure baby has cap, socks, and nappy, and is undressed.	
• Procedure: – Ask the mother to sit comfortably on the chair. – Place baby prone on the mother's chest in an upright position in between the breasts. – Ensure skin-to-skin contact. – Keep baby in frog-like position (arms and legs flexed). – Turn baby's head to one side so airway is open. – Support baby's head with mother's hand. – Support baby's bottom using appropriate sling or binder. – Cover mother and baby with blanket or shawl. – Plan to provide KMC at least for an hour.	
• Monitor: – Check the baby's color, position, and breathing. – Inform mother of danger signs.	
Ensure baby is fed on demand.	

12. HAND WASH

Steps	*Tick*
Ensure there are no watch, thread, rings, or bangles on hands.	
Wet hands under running water. Apply soap.	
• Vigorously rub hands on both sides in following manner: – Palms, fingers, and web spaces – Back of hands – Knuckles – Thumbs – Fingertips and creases – Wrist and forearm up to the elbow	
Rinse hands in running water.	
Allow hands to air-dry ensuring no touch and hands remain above waist level.	

CHAPTER 6.2

Drugs

1.

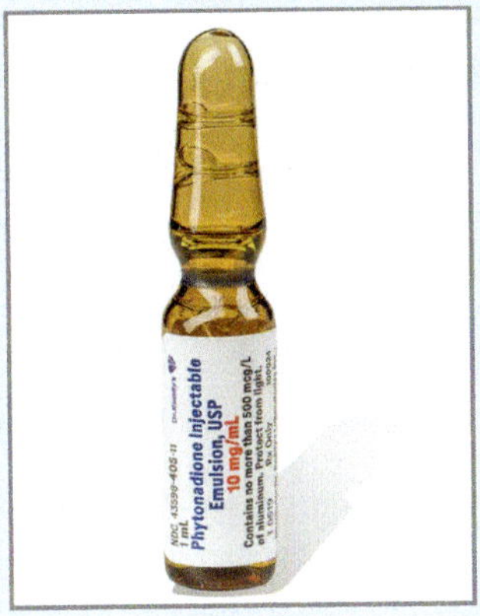

a. What is the dose for prevention of vitamin K deficiency bleeding (VKDB) based on weight as per Government of India guidelines?
b. Why is intramuscular (IM) route preferred over oral route in neonates?
c. Why is this form of vitamin K preferred over menadione?
d. In which type of VKDB is intracranial hemorrhage most common?
e. Name four conditions where you need to supplement postnatally.
f. Name coagulation factors dependent on vitamin K.

Ans.

a. IM, 0.5 mg for <1,000 g, 1 mg if weight >1,000 g.
b. Oral route needs periodic dosages unlike IM dose which is single.
c. Menadione displaces bilirubin from albumin thereby predisposing to bilirubin encephalopathy hence vitamin K_1 is preferred.
d. Late VKDB
e. Cholestasis syndromes, malabsorption syndrome, cystic fibrosis, prolonged antibiotics, alpha 1 antitrypsin deficiency, chronic diarrhea
f. Factors II, VII, IX, and X

2.

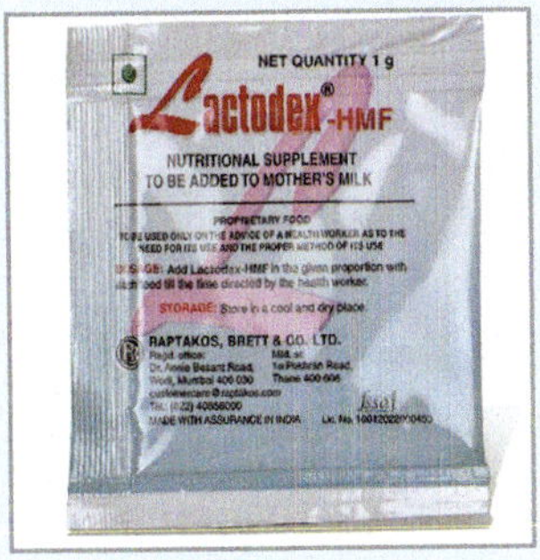

a. At what volume of milk intake is it recommended?
b. At what age is it stopped?
c. How do you assess for protein adequacy biochemically?
d. Name four potential side effects.
e. Name two supplements which should be stopped if the baby is on human milk fortifier (HMF)?

Ans.

a. 100 cc/kg/day
b. 40 weeks of postnatal age or when the baby is on full and direct breast feeds
c. Blood urea nitrogen (BUN) values (if <10 mg/dL suggests increasing protein)
d. Nosocomial infection, under- or overdilution, feed intolerance, necrotizing enterocolitis (NEC)
e. Vitamin D, iron, multivitamin drops

3.

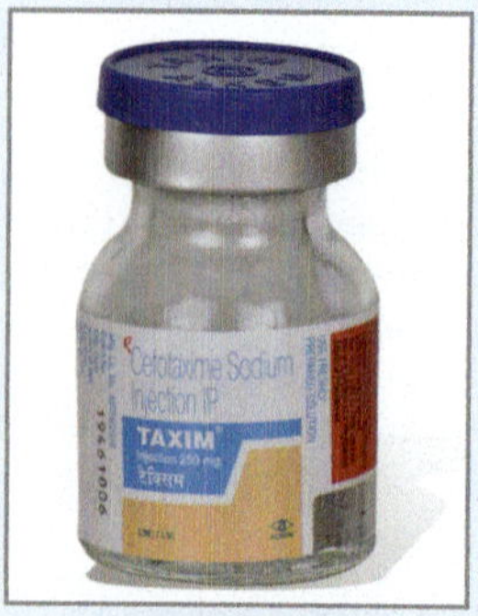

a. Name four disadvantages of its empiric use.
b. When is its use preferred empirically?
c. On what two factors is its dose based in sepsis?
d. With what solution is the injection diluted?
e. What solution is used to flush before and after drug delivery?
f. What precaution is used with coadministration of aminoglycoside?

Ans.

a. Increased risk of multidrug resistance, late-onset sepsis, NEC, invasive fungal infection and death
b. Suspected meningitis
c. Postnatal age and gestation
d. Water for injection
e. 0.9% sodium chloride
f. Separate aminoglycoside administration by at least 1 hour.

4.

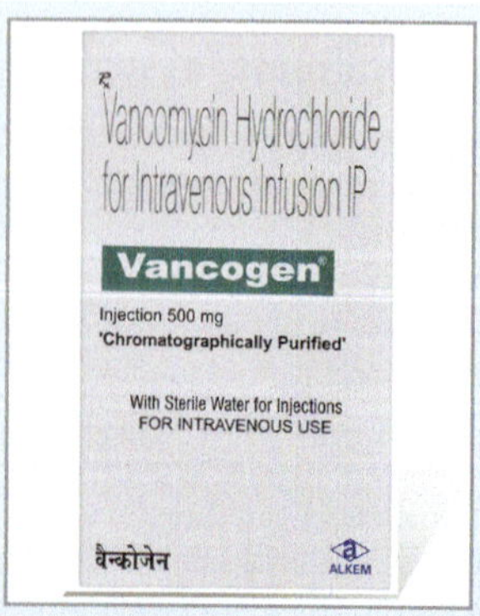

a. Name two neonatal factors on which the dose is based.
b. Name two drugs incompatible (Y site) with it.
c. Why is the drug administered as an infusion over few hours?
d. With anaphylactoid reaction, what two immediate measures should be taken?
e. Name four concomitant factors, which may predispose to nephrotoxicity.
f. What parameter should be monitored daily and weekly with this drug?

Ans.

a. Gestation and postnatal age
b. Potassium phosphate, heparin, piperacillin/tazobactam, hydrocortisone, ceftazidime, furosemide, methylprednisolone, and phenytoin
c. To avoid red man syndrome, viz., erythematous reactions, flushing, tachycardia, and hypotension
d. Pause therapy, give diphenhydramine, resume infusion over longer period once symptoms resolve
e. Drug therapy duration >7 days, vasopressors, aminoglycosides, frusemide, piperacillin/tazobactam
f. Urine output daily and BUN/serum creatinine weekly

5.

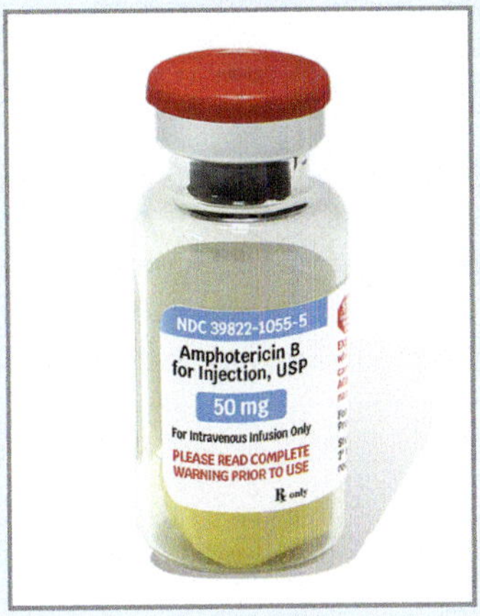

a. What solution is used for dilution? What buffer is added to diluted drug for administration?
b. Where is it stored in neonatal intensive care unit (NICU)? Name two similar drugs for storage.
c. Why is sodium chloride not used for its reconstitution?
d. What do you flush the line before and after its administration?
e. Over what period of time is the infusion administered? What is the hazard of rapid infusion?
f. In which fungal infection is its use not recommended?
g. When do you consider discontinuation with renal impairment?

Ans.

a. Water for injection, glucose
b. 2°C–8°C in refrigerator; other drugs requiring refrigeration are surfactant, adenosine, insulin, amoxicillin-clavulanate, prostaglandin preparation
c. Causes precipitation
d. 5% glucose
e. Over 4–6 hours, rapid infusion may cause cardiotoxicity, hyperkalemia, and arrhythmia
f. Candiduria, renal fungal balls
g. If serum creatinine is double the normal value

6.

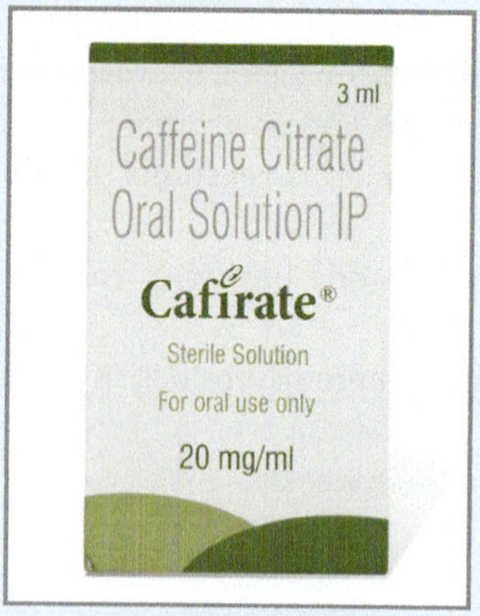

a. How is diagnosis of apnea of prematurity confirmed?
b. Name three benefits of starting early therapy (<3 days).
c. Name four common features of accidental drug overdose.
d. What is its effect on patent ductus arteriosus (PDA)?
e. What is its effect on retinopathy of prematurity (ROP)?
f. What is its effect on NEC?
g. Name two contraindications.
h. How long does it take for complete action to start after the loading dose?

Ans.

a. Diagnosis of exclusion
b. Less incidence of bronchopulmonary dysplasia (BPD), less treatment of PDA, and shorter duration of mechanical ventilation
c. Tachycardia, tachypnea, agitation, irritability, tremor, hypertonia, and tonic-clonic movements
d. Less likely to require pharmacological treatment and surgical ligation for PDA
e. Fewer infants with severe ROP
f. No increment in NEC
g. Concomitant xanthine therapy, gastrointestinal (GI) bleed, liver or renal dysfunction
h. 5–6 days

7.

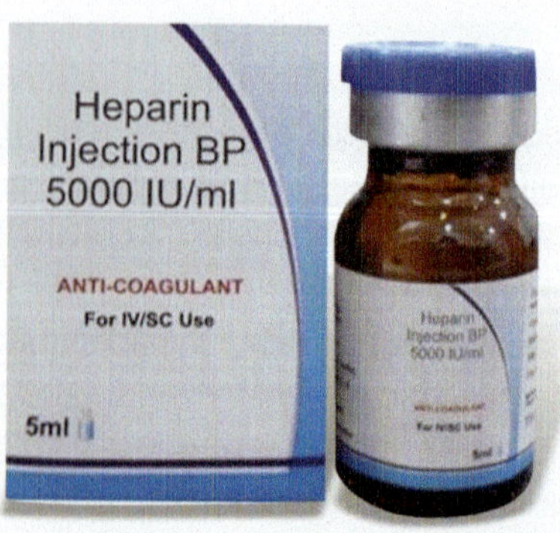

a. What dilution is required to flush ABG syringe?
b. What is the dilution effect on ABG?
c. What is the concentration effect on ABG?
d. Name two contraindications.
e. Name two concomitant drugs, which increase bleeding tendency.
f. Name its antidote.
g. Name two drugs incompatible (Y site) with its use.

Ans.

a. 100 IU/mL
b. Dilution effect of heparin in syringe may cause fall in partial pressure of carbon dioxide (pCO_2) and bicarbonate concentration.
c. Concentrated heparin may result in an increase in pCO_2 and reduction in pH.
d. Uncontrolled bleeding, intraventricular hemorrhage, GI hemorrhage, thrombocytopenia (<50, 000), severe hypertension
e. Paracetamol, nonsteroid anti-inflammatory drugs, alprostadil
f. Protamine sulfate
g. Benzylpenicillin, ciprofloxacin, dobutamine, erythromycin, gentamicin, ketamine

8.

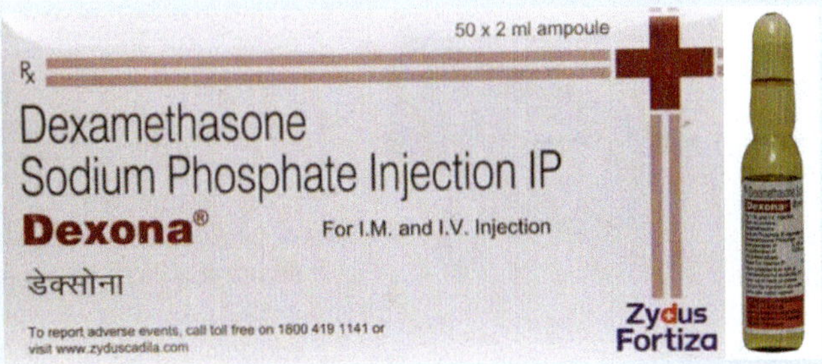

a. Why is it preferred over betamethasone in India for preterm labor?
b. What is its dose for prevention of respiratory distress syndrome (RDS)?
c. Name an absolute contraindication.
d. When does its action begin and how long does it last?
e. When is repeat course advisable?

Ans.

a. Betamethasone acetate/phosphate is not available in India.
b. 6 mg, 12 hourly × 4 doses, IM in all mothers with threatened preterm labor
c. Chorioamnionitis in mother
d. 24 hours after the course and lasts for 7 days
e. In women in whom preterm birth is expected within 72 hours and who have had one course of corticosteroids more than a week ago.

CHAPTER

6.3

Instruments

1.

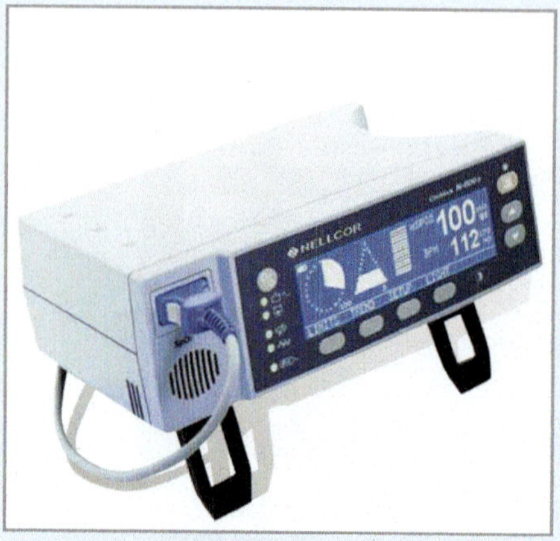

a. On what principle does it work?
b. Name four drawbacks of this instrument.
c. Name four factors which move the oxygen dissociation curve to the right.
d. Which technology is preferred in the delivery room for measurement of this vital?
e. What does low peripheral oxygen saturation (SpO_2) but normal partial pressure of oxygen (PaO_2) suggest?
f. How does one ensure the displayed SpO_2 is correct?
g. What congenital heart defects (CHDs) are identified by pulse oximeter screening?

Ans.

a. Identify difference between absorption of infrared and red light and the microprocessor calculates the ratio between oxygen rich and oxygen poor hemoglobin. It works on Beer–Lambert law.
b. Inappropriate measurement with movements, skin pigmentation, hypothermia, shock, phototherapy, does not measure oxygen content, oxygen delivery, and oxygen consumption
c. Hyperthermia, hypercarbia, acidosis, and blood transfusion
d. Signal extraction technology
e. Abnormal hemoglobin (methemoglobinemia)
f. Heart rate correlates with auscultation or with electrocardiogram (ECG), pulse wave form is uniform.
g. d-transposition of the great arteries (d-TGA), critical pulmonary stenosis, total anomalous pulmonary venous connection (TAPVC), pulmonary atresia, truncus arteriosus, single ventricle, hypoplastic left heart syndrome

2.

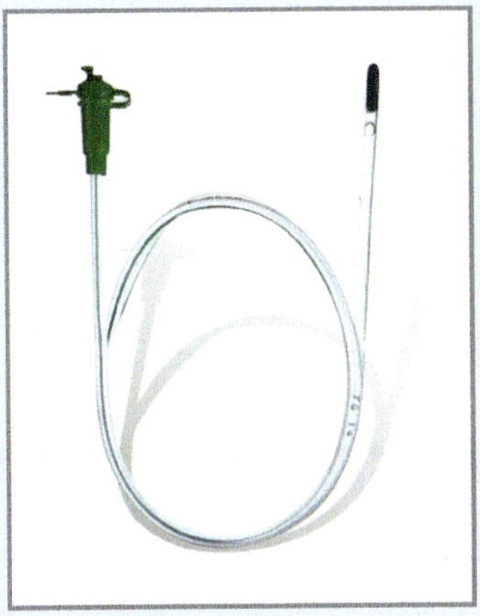

a. How do you measure the depth of insertion for orogastric tube?
b. Name two non-nutritional indications for its use.
c. Name two respiratory care indications.
d. Name four markers for its appropriate placement.
e. What does its position in thorax imply?
f. What does its position away from midline imply?
g. Name two surgical conditions where its use is recommended at the earliest.
h. Name two pain relief measures prior to insertion.
i. Name four risks associated with its use?

Ans.

a. Tip of the *nose* to the *ear* lobe to a point midway between *xiphoid* and umbilicus (NEX)
b. Gastric lavage, medication administration, check patency of nostrils
c. Deflate stomach during prolonged bag and mask ventilation, adjunct to continuous positive airway pressure (CPAP) therapy
d. Aspiration of gastric content, hissing sound over stomach on flushing with air, gastric aspirate check with pH strip (≤6), X-ray and well-being of the baby
e. Diaphragmatic hernia
f. Space occupying lesion in thorax
g. Abdominal wall defects (e.g., exomphalos), suspected intestinal obstruction
h. Stroking, holding and talking to the baby, massage, oral breast milk, sucrose
i. Displacement, aspiration, pain, mucosal or skin injury

3.

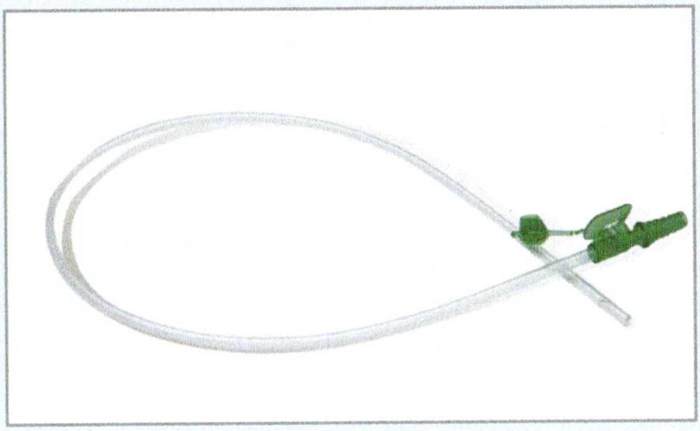

a. Name its four clinical uses during ventilation.
b. What is the advantage of using this type of catheter over the conventional one?
c. What is the maximum pressure limit during its use?
d. Name four advantages of closed suction.
e. Name four risks associated with its use.

Ans.

a. Desaturation, visible secretions, chest retractions, sudden deterioration, minimal or no chest wall movement, decreased breath sounds
b. Thumb-operated suction allows for ease of applying pressure.
c. 80–100 mm Hg
d. Prevents lung de-recruitment, reduces contamination of environmental pathogens, reduces viral/bacterial contamination, protects staff from accidental exposure to secretions, minimizes risk of ventilator associated pneumonia
e. Hypoxia, bradycardia, mucosal injury, apnea, airleak, atelectasis

4.

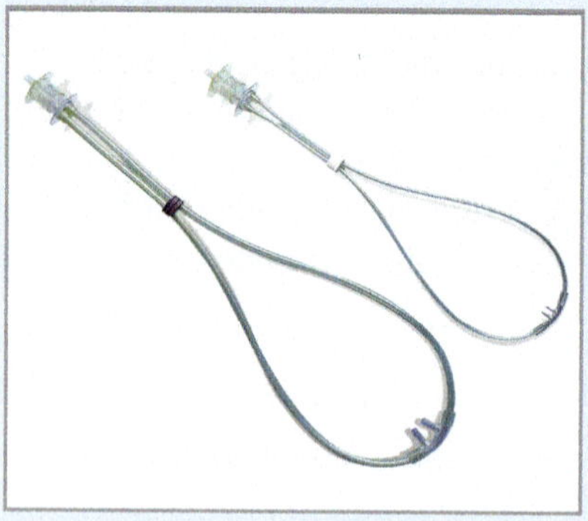

a. Identify.
b. Name two indications for its use.
c. Name the maximum flow and oxygen that can be delivered with it.
d. Preferably below what gestation is its use not recommended?
e. What should be the prong size?
f. Name four contraindications for its use.
g. Name four risks associated with its use.
h. What adjunct measure should be taken with its use?
i. What are main differences between nasal prongs used for CPAP versus those used for high-flow nasal cannula (HFNC)?

Ans.

a. Ram cannula
b. Nasal interface for CPAP and nasal noninvasive ventilation (NIV)
c. 8 L/min, 60% oxygen
d. 28 weeks and <1,000 g
e. Not more than 80% diameter of the nostrils
f. Severe respiratory distress, orofacial anomaly (cleft lip/palate, nasal atresia), shock, congenital diaphragmatic hernia, tracheoesophageal fistula, air leak
g. Nasal trauma, gastric distention, hypoxia due to block or displacement, skin injury
h. Orogastric tube placement

i. The prongs are wide, snuggly fitting in CPAP while narrow, tapered, and loosely fitting (<50% of nostrils) for HFNC.

5.

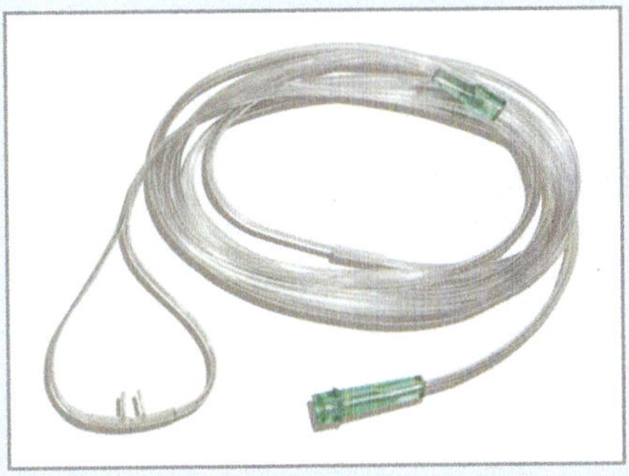

a. Identify.
b. Name two indications for its use.
c. Name the maximum flow and oxygen that can be delivered with it.
d. What recommended water level in the oxygen jar when using this?
e. What is the target oxygen saturation with its use?

Ans.

a. Low-flow nasal cannula
b. For mild respiratory distress, step down from CPAP or HFNC
c. 2 L/min, 30%
d. Do not use water in the oxygen jar when flow rates are <2 L/min
e. 91%–95%

6.

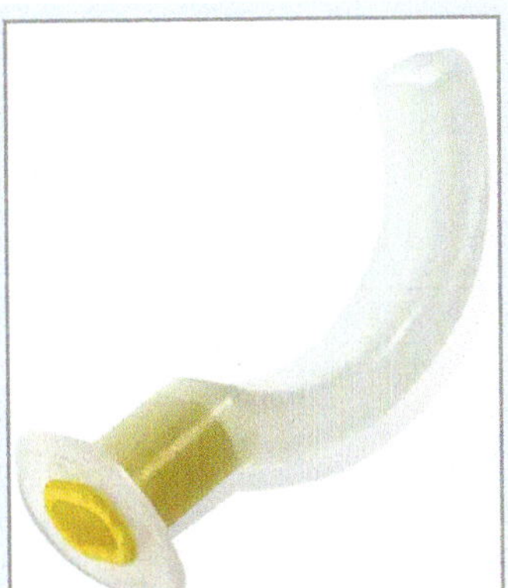

a. Identify.
b. How do you decide the depth of insertion?
c. Name a contraindication for its use.
d. Name an indication.
e. What is the technique of insertion?

Ans.

a. Oropharyngeal airway
b. From the center of the incisors to the angle of the mandible with the convex side up
c. Conscious patient with an intact gag reflex, nasal fracture, or active nose bleeding
d. Upper airway obstruction, e.g., bilateral choanal atresia, tongue causing obstruction, severe Pierre Robin sequence

e. Raise the shoulder with a roll, inserted under direct vision with the concave side up and gently rotate 180°.

7.

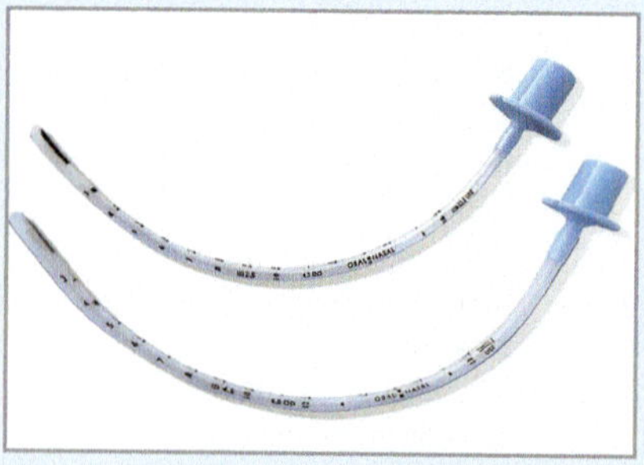

a. Name the most reliable way to decide the tube depth.
b. How do you decide the depth of insertion in emergency for oral intubation?
c. Why un-cuffed tubes are preferred?
d. Name two elective intubation uses.
e. Why is weight-based insertion formula no longer used?
f. Name two reasons why endotracheal (ET) tube is cut at 3–4 cm beyond the lips.
g. Name the gold standard to confirm right position of the tip.

Ans.

a. Based on gestation
b. Tip of nose to the tragus of the ear plus 1 cm for oral intubation
c. To avoid edema or pressure changes at the cricoid ring
d. Prenatal diagnosis of diaphragmatic hernia, surfactant administration, prior to major surgery, prolonged bag and mask ventilation, prior to transport
e. Overestimates insertion depth in extremely low birth weight (ELBW) infants
f. Minimize resistance, minimize dead space, prevent kinking of tube
g. X-ray chest—ET tip should be 1 cm above carina (T2–T3)

8.

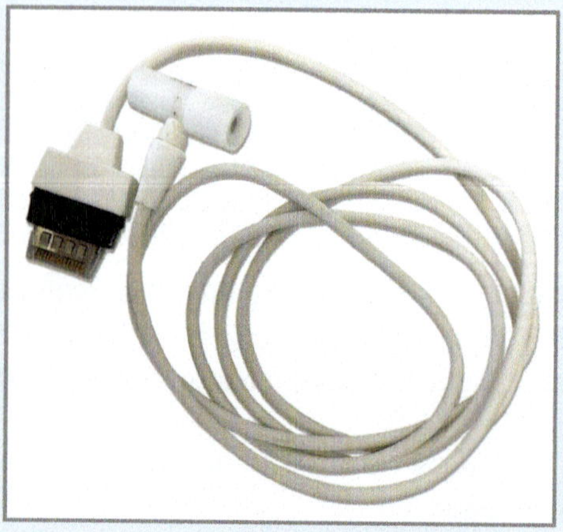

a. Identify.
b. Name four benefits of its use.
c. Name four different ways by such devices work.
d. Name two problems associated with it.
e. What mode does the ventilator deliver in absence of this?

Ans.

a. Flow sensor
b. Allows accurate measurement of pressure, flows, tidal volumes, respiratory mechanics (compliance, resistance); facilitates triggering, volume targeting, and flow cycling
c. Abdominal motion, thoracic impedance, airway flow, airway pressure
d. Need to set trigger threshold, autocycling, artefactual triggering
e. Conventional or intermittent mandatory ventilation

9.

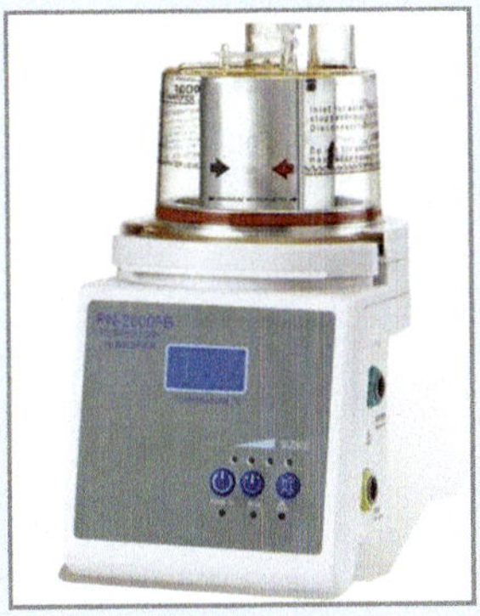

a. Identify.
b. What settings of temperature and humidity is used in the newborn?
c. How do you know humidification is adequate?
d. Name four problems if it malfunctions.
e. What is the unit for absolute humidity?

Ans.

a. Servo humidifier
b. Temperature of 37°C and 100% relative humidity
c. No condensation in the inspiratory circuit, minimal condensation in expiratory circuit, display's temperature of 37°C on the monitor
d. Water trapping in circuit, tube block, aspiration pneumonia, disruption of respiratory epithelium, bronchospasm, atelectasis, autotriggering
e. Grams per cubic meter of air

10.

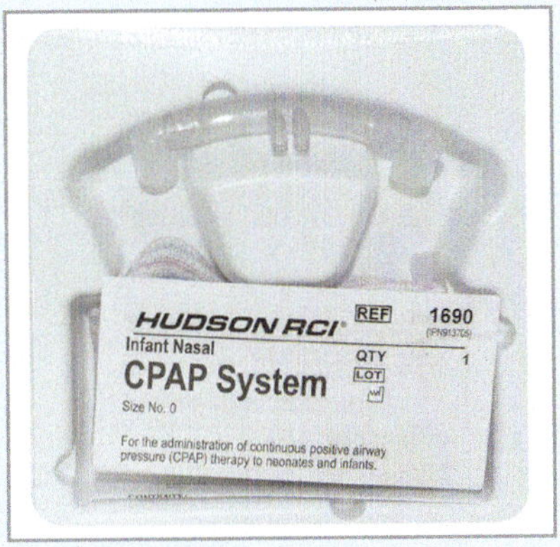

a. How do you decide on prong size and placement?
b. How do you ensure the cap is appropriately placed?
c. How do you judge adequacy of CPAP clinically?
d. Name two contraindications for its use?
e. In case of nasal injury how do you continue with CPAP?

Ans.

a. The prong should be snugly fitting the nostril with a gap of at least 2 mm from the nasal septum/columella.
b. Cap should be snugly fitting and covering both the ears.
c. Comfortable baby, regular breathing with no retractions or grunt, bilateral bubbling sound in the chest, oxygen saturation 91–95%.
d. Orofacial anomaly, poor or absent respiratory drive, shock, congenital diaphragmatic hernia, tracheoesophageal fistula
e. Using nasal mask

SECTION 7

Counseling

7. Counseling
   - 7.1 Counseling—Long-term Drug Therapy, e.g., Levothyroxine
   - 7.2 Dealing with Treatment Options, e.g., Jaundice: Phototherapy versus Exchange Transfusion
   - 7.3 Calling a Colleague for Transfer of Patient—SBARR Protocol
   - 7.4 Communicating Sad/Bad News—SPIKES Protocol
   - 7.5 Disclosing Medical Error, Sudden Deterioration or Sudden Death—CONES Protocol
   - 7.6 Challenging Emotional Encounters with Family—BUSTER Protocol
   - 7.7 Counsel Mother in Postnatal Ward on Exclusive Breastfeeding Advantages

CHAPTER 7

Counseling

7.1 COUNSELING—LONG-TERM DRUG THERAPY, E.G., LEVOTHYROXINE

	Tick here
Initiating session: • Introduces self, greets parents • Makes parents comfortable by inviting to sit • Ensures private area with no distractions • Is attentive. Informs purpose of visit	
Gathering information: • Start with an open ended Qs: *What do you know about the babies treatment?* • Enquires about the parental concerns, ideas about the treatment?	
Explanation: • *How treatment works?* Thyroxine is a synthetic preparation mimicking natural hormone. It is meant to replace and overcome thyroid hormone deficiency which the baby is suffering from. This will help bring babies thyroid activity back to normal	
• *How to take drug?* Once daily, early morning, same time every day, crush and mix with mother's milk, and give by dropper or syringe. Ensure iron, multivitamins, and calcium are supplemented at another time to avoid errors in thyroid drug absorption	
• *What to monitor?* Monitor serum thyroid-stimulating hormone (TSH) levels periodically as advised. The dose will be adjusted based on your babies TSH levels. It takes 4–6 weeks for dose change effects to take place	
• *What are the side effects?* Side effects are rare. High dose may cause diarrhea, vomiting, and low dose may cause constipation	
Summarizes key points: • Don't miss the dose • Don't stop drug on own • Long-term therapy is must • Monitor labs as advised to adjust dose • Giving right dose at the right time will help maintain your babies, growth and brain development	

Contd...

Contd...

	Tick here
Building the relationship: • Listens attentively without interruption • Accept parent/s views and feelings nonjudgmentally • Acknowledges parent/s feelings, emotions, and uncertainty • Provides support, hope, and deals sensitively • Clarifies information and summarizes periodically • Uses simple language • Maintain eye contact except when the patient becomes upset • Provides options, choices and is nondirective • Uses pictures, graphs, or illustration • Do not respond to phone calls, pagers, but if you must apologize to the parent before answering • Involves patient/s in care discussions	
Closing the session: • Confirms parental understanding • Asks for any questions, concerns, or clarifications • Responds to parental queries • Ascertain level of involvement parent/s wishes in decision making • Informs repeat consult to meet their requirement • Schedules next consult, when and how to seek help • Confirms parent/s agree and are comfortable with plan • Thanks the parent/s	

7.2 DEALING WITH TREATMENT OPTIONS, E.G., JAUNDICE: PHOTOTHERAPY VERSUS EXCHANGE TRANSFUSION

Use format as given in first example for initiating session, gathering information, building relationships, and closing the session.

Use the following format for "explanation".

Q's	*Phototherapy*	*Exchange transfusion*
Why is this treatment offered?	If the bilirubin levels in blood increases to a certain level there is a possible risk of brain damage. This risk can be reduced by lowering the bilirubin values using special light for treatment	If there is rapid rise in bilirubin values despite phototherapy then the bilirubin levels can be brought down by replacing baby's blood by this procedure
What does this treatment involve?	Baby is placed naked with eyes covered under special light source and blood is monitored periodically to see the effectiveness. The mother can frequently visit, hold, and feed the baby	The baby's blood is cross matched with donor blood in the blood bank. Through umbilical access, a fixed amount of baby's blood is withdrawn and replaced by donor blood for over 1 hour. The procedure is performed in neonatal intensive care unit (NICU) under strict asepsis and closely monitored. Blood sample is sent postprocedure to see effectiveness of therapy

Contd...

Contd…

Q's	*Phototherapy*	*Exchange transfusion*
How long will it take for the treatment to work?	This depends on the jaundice cause, severity and timing of therapy. In majority, the bilirubin values start falling by 12–24 hours of initiating therapy. The therapy needs to be continued till we reach safe bilirubin values	This depends on the jaundice cause, severity and timing of therapy. Postprocedure the baby is initiated on continuous phototherapy. In majority the bilirubin values start falling by 12–24 hours post procedure
What are the risks of this treatment?	In majority the therapy is without any major risk. Risk of serious harm is rare	As with any procedure there may be rare event of death (<1 per 100 or <1%), 1% may require repeat procedure for rising bilirubin
What are the side effects of this?	There may be rash, diarrhea, or fever	The side effects may be infection or bleeding (1–2 per 100, i.e., 1 or 2%), decrease in calcium, change in electrolytes or heart rhythm
How long will it take to recover?	This depends on the cause of jaundice. We shall monitor bilirubin values periodically and keep you informed. The baby is fit for discharge once we reach safe bilirubin levels	The baby is shifted to phototherapy once the procedure is over. The baby's bilirubin values are checked periodically and baby is fit for discharge once we reach safe bilirubin levels

7.3 CALLING A COLLEAGUE FOR TRANSFER OF PATIENT—SBARR PROTOCOL

S	*Situation*: • I am Dr X from ward Y from hospital Z • I am calling for patient XX who is X day's old • The reason I am calling is the baby is suspected to have a surgical condition and needs surgery ASAP
B	*Background*: • Patient XY was a normal delivery born on x.x.xx. He was well till few hours back when he was noticed to have frothing at mouth • We could not insert feeding tube per mouth. There is coiling of tube on X-ray taken. We suspect surgical cause • The baby is x gestation, weights xx, and has no associated anomalies
A	*Assessment*: • The baby's vital parameters are stable as of now viz HR 120 beats/min, RR 45 breaths/min, SpO_2 92% in room air • In view of suspected surgical condition, I have kept the baby nil-by-mouth, started on intravenous (IV) fluids, nursed the baby in prone position with frequent oral suction

Contd…

Contd...

R	*Recommendation:* In view of surgical condition, I need to transfer the baby for surgical management to your hospital
R	*Readback:* • The listener responds • Ok. So, we agree to the plan for immediate transfer of this baby to your hospital. We shall do the needful at earliest. Thank you

7.4 COMMUNICATING SAD/BAD NEWS—SPIKES PROTOCOL

S	*Setup*: • Introduce self • Ensure private area with no distractions • Make the parent/s, relative/s comfortable by inviting to sit • Remain attentive, give undivided attention • Prepare for what to say and anticipate the patient/family reaction • Have the key people in the room • Be calm. Take care not to be overcome by your own emotions
P	*Perception*: • Start with open ended Q—*"Can you tell me more about your baby's concerns?" "Tell me what you understand about your condition so far." "What did the other doctors tell you?" "I'd like to be sure we are on the same page with understanding your condition, so can you tell me..."* • Know the parent/s, relative/s perception of illness so far • Assess the patient and family members' level of understanding • Take note of discrepancies in the patient's understanding and what is actually true • Watch for signs of denial • Accept parent/s views and feelings nonjudgmentally
I	*Invite*: • Informs purpose of meeting. *"Today my plan is to discuss...is that okay?"* • Ask the parent/s if they want to know the details of the medical condition/ treatment. *"I'd like to go over the results, would that be ok?"* • Invite parents to care decision making • Establish how much they wish to be involved in decision making
K	*Knowledge transfer*: • Use name of the baby • Inform the present critical condition of the baby • Inform all possible care being provided • Inform despite all best care, poor response to therapy • Inform possible outcomes • Present the information in small chunks. • After each chunk, verify the patient's understanding. *"Are you with me so far?* • Ask for any questions, concerns or clarifications • Respond to parental queries • Use simple, nontechnical words • Pause periodically for information to sink in

Contd...

Contd...

E	*Empathy*: • Verbally acknowledge the feelings, emotions, and uncertainty • Identify the emotion. Identify the cause of the emotion • Respond by showing you have made the connection between the emotion and the cause *"I can see you weren't expecting this." "Most people would be upset finding this out." ....."I'm sorry this has happened and I understand how it would make you feel that way."......"I hear what you're saying. That must have been very difficult."....."I get your point. It was obviously very upsetting"* • Provide unrestricted time • Listen attentively without interruption • Provide support, hope and deals sensitively • Maintain eye contact except when the patient becomes upset • Avoid phrases such as: *"I know how you feel."......"I feel your pain."......"It's going to be alright"*
S	*Summarize*: • Repeat key information slowly and clearly • Ask if the parent/s has any other questions for you • If there are no Q or if you don't have time for further questions, suggest that they can be addressed at the next appointment • Reassure parent/s that you are and will be available to help • Confirm parent/s agree and are comfortable with plan • Thank the parent/s

7.5 DISCLOSING MEDICAL ERROR, SUDDEN DETERIORATION OR SUDDEN DEATH—CONES PROTOCOL

C	*Context*: • Plan what you'll say and anticipate how the parent/family might react • Choose a quiet, private setting for the conversation • Sit down, stay calm, and maintain eye contact
O	*Opening*: Alert the parent/family member of important news. • *I have some important news to share about your baby's condition"* • *"This is challenging, but I need to give you some important information"* • *"I need to discuss your baby's condition with you"* • *"Thank you for coming in. I need to update you on what's happening with your baby*
N	*Narrative approach*: • Explain chronology of events: *"To recap, your baby came in on..." "We then administered... but saw minimal improvement."..... "Last night, we... and I've just learned that..."......"In summary, she received an excessive amount of drug"* • Emphasize you are investigating how the error occurred: *"We've initiated an investigation into how this error happened, and I aim to provide clear answers by the end of today."…. "I hope that by the end of the day, we will see some improvement"* • Offer apology: *"I sincerely apologize for this situation"*

Contd...

Contd...

E	*Emotions*: • Verbally acknowledge the feelings, emotions, and uncertainty. • Identify the emotion. Identify the cause of the emotion. Respond by showing you have made the connection between the emotion and the cause. *"I can see you weren't expecting this."... "I know it is upsetting for you and it's awful for me too."... "It is very rare, but it does happen and I am sorry to say that it did"* • Avoid false hope, assurance or outcome • Avoid phrases such as: *"I know how you feel."......"I feel your pain."......"It's going to be alright"*
S	*Summarize*: • Repeat key information slowly and clearly • Let the parent/s know the situation is a priority *"I am the doctor responsible for your baby so it is important that I found out what happened."........"I can guarantee we will do our best."...."Here is what I propose we do."....."Let's meet at the end of today or I can call you when I know more"* • Reassure parent/s that you are and will be available to help • Thank the parent/s

7.6 CHALLENGING EMOTIONAL ENCOUNTERS WITH FAMILY—BUSTER PROTOCOL

B	*Be prepared*: • Anticipate that both you and the other person may experience strong emotions • Prepare a strategy for delivering difficult news • Be aware of your own thoughts and feelings, as this awareness can enhance your communication • Practice self-regulation to manage your emotions, especially when provoked • Try to transform conflicts into productive conversations • Recognize when it is best to postpone the discussion if emotions are running too high
U	*Use nonjudgmental listening*: • Maintain eye contact throughout the conversation • Listen attentively without interrupting, only using clarifying questions and paraphrasing to ensure understanding. *"Let me confirm if I understand correctly..." "What I'm hearing is..."* • Set aside your own agenda until the other person has finished speaking • Refrain from minimizing the seriousness of the situation *"I understand this is very difficult, and it may be more challenging than we initially anticipated*
S	*Six second rule*: • When you start to feel intense emotions, particularly in response to anger or blame, take at least 6 seconds or longer to calm yourself before responding • Collect your thoughts and use techniques like "Tell me more" or respond with empathy and validation

Contd...

Contd...

T	*"Tell me more" statements*: Encourage the person to elaborate on their thoughts. • "Can you share more about your problem?" • "What occurred after that?" • "What additional concerns do you have?"
E	*Empathize and validate*: Acknowledge emotions by empathizing: • I can tell this was unexpected for you" • "This is a tough conversation, isn't it?" • "I understand how stressful this situation is" • "It must be challenging to come here every week" • "I see how difficult this is for you"
R	*Respond with a wish statement*: Let the other person know you hear them and acknowledge that the goal may be desirable, but... • "I wish I could share better news with you..." • "I wish I didn't have to deliver this message..." • "I wish we had a more effective treatment available • "I wish things had turned out differently"

7.7 COUNSEL MOTHER IN POSTNATAL WARD ON EXCLUSIVE BREASTFEEDING ADVANTAGES

	Tick here
Initiating session: • Introduces self, greets mother • Makes mother comfortable by inviting to sit • Ensures private area with no distractions • Is attentive. Informs purpose of visit	
Gathering information: • Start with an open ended Q: *What has been your past breastfeeding experience? What are the benefits of breastfeeding for your baby?* • Enquires about the parental concerns, ideas about the breastfeeding • Appreciates her response • Remains nonjudgmental	
Explanation: • *How breastfeeding works?* Breastfeeding is a complete food for your baby. It is nature's gift to meet the complete nutritional, immunological, emotional, and spiritual requirements of your baby. Your baby when breastfed exclusively has optimum physical growth, brain development, lesser infections, lesser allergies, lesser risk of pneumonia, higher IQ, and lesser risks of adult-onset disorders such as obesity, hypertension, and heart disease. Breast milk is available on demand, easy to digest, helps bonding and protects you from bleeding and pregnancy • *How to practice breastfeeding?* You should feed only your milk and nothing else—no water, ghutti, gripe water, honey, or any top milk. Baby needs to be fed on demand, every 4–6 hours as required, initiating with one breast and thereafter shifting to another. You should provide only your milk during first 6 months of age—no water or anything else	

Contd...

Contd...

	Tick here
• *What to monitor?* A baby when breastfeeds adequately has clear, colorless urine, and passes stools frequently. Baby appears to be contended after feed and sleeps peacefully	
Summarizes key point: • Breast milk is the best choice of feeding • Breastfeeding must be exclusive • Breastfeeding should be on demand • Breastfeeding ensures optimal growth and development for the baby. It is also beneficial to mother's wellbeing	
Building the relationship: • Listens attentively without interruption • Accept mother's views and feelings nonjudgmentally • Acknowledges mother's feelings, emotions, and uncertainty • Clarifies information and summarizes periodically • Uses simple language • Maintain eye contact • Uses pictures, graphs or illustration • Do not respond to phone calls, pagers, but if you must apologize to the parent before answering • Involves mother in care discussions	
Closing the session: • Confirms mothers understanding • Asks for any questions, concerns or clarifications • Responds to parental queries • Informs repeat consult to meet their requirement • Schedules next consult, when and how to seek help • Confirms mother agree and are comfortable with plan • Thanks the mother	

SECTION 8

Miscellaneous

CHAPTER 8.1

Miscellaneous OSCE

Q1. Identify the logo.

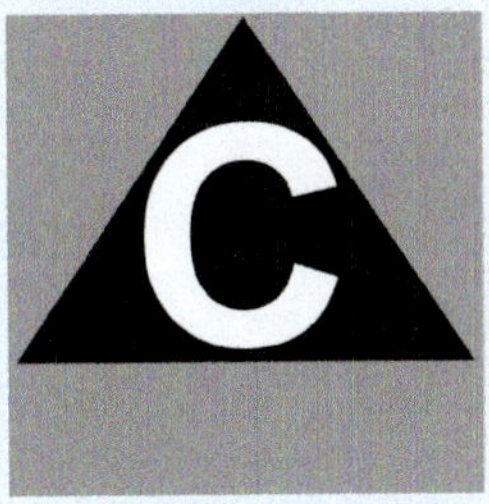

Cytotoxic

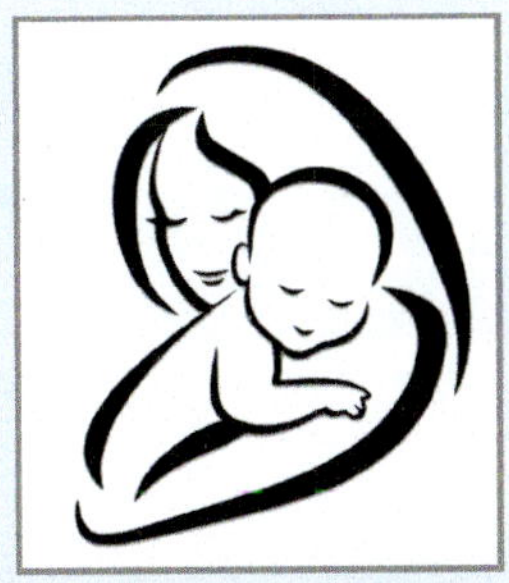

Janani Suraksha Yojana (JSY)

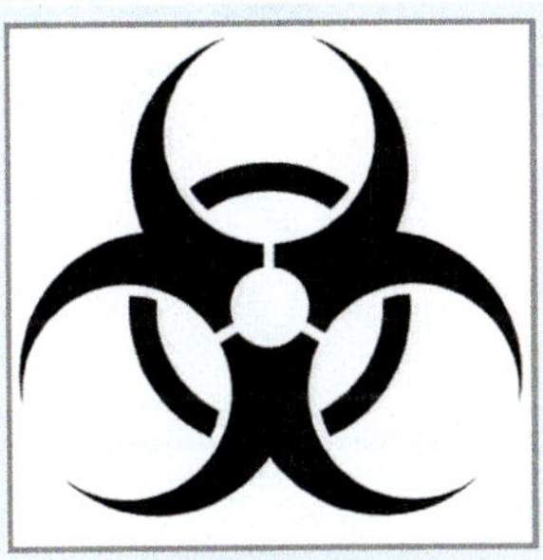

Biohazard

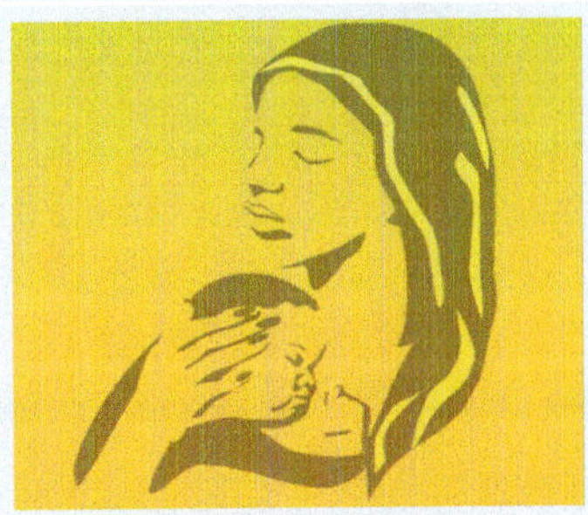

Janani Shishu Suraksha Karyakram (JSSK)

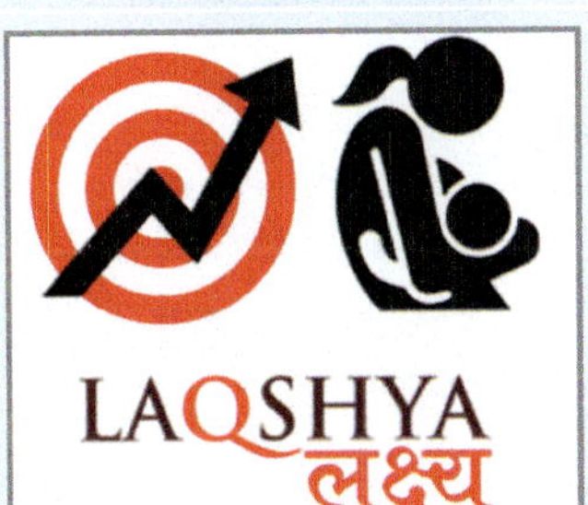

Labor Room Quality Improvement Initiative

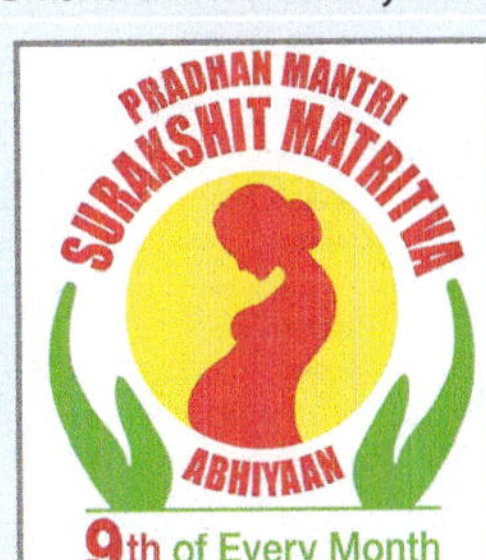

Pradhan Mantri Surakshit Matritva Abhiyaan (PMSMA)

Surkashit Matrutva Ashwasan (SUMAN)

Pradhan Mantra Matru Vandana Yojana (PMMVY)

Integrated Government Online Training

National Health Mission (NHM)

India Newborn Action Plan (INAP)

Human Milk Bank Association

Cochrane

Mothers' Absolute Affection (MAA)

World Health Organization (WHO)

Mission Indradhanush

United Nations Children's Fund (UNICEF)

Rashtriya Bal Swasthya Karyakram (RBSK)

Q2. Match the National program with its objective.

Program	*Objective*
1. Janani Suraksha Yojana (JSY)	a. To increase the number of institutional deliveries by providing cashless service benefits to all pregnant women and sick infants admitted in public health institutions
2. Janani Shishu Suraksha Karyakram (JSSK)	b. To improve perinatal care by providing fixed day assured, comprehensive, and quality antenatal care universally to all pregnant women
3. Pradhan Mantri Surakshit Matritva Abhiyan (PMSMA)	c. To reduce maternal and neonatal mortality by promoting institutional delivery among pregnant women
4. Pradhan Mantri Matru Vandana Yojana (PMMVY)	d. To provide partial compensation for the wage loss in terms of cash incentive so that the pregnant woman can take adequate rest before and after delivery of the first living child
5. Labor room Quality Improvement Initiative (LaQshya)	e. To empower the healthcare providers with the skills to manage neonatal and childhood illnesses at the community as well as facility level, by ensuring standard case management of major causes of neonatal and childhood morbidity and mortality

Contd...

Contd...

Program	*Objective*
6. Facility-based Integrated Management of Neonatal and Childhood Illness (F-IMNCI)	f. To reduce infant mortality by ensuring availability of healthcare personnel trained in basic essential newborn care and neonatal resuscitation at every delivery point
7. Navjat Shishu Suraksha Karyakram (NSSK)	g. To provide respectful maternity care (RMC) to all pregnant women attending public health facilities
8. Facility Based Newborn Care (FBNC)	h. To reduce neonatal mortality by providing facility based newborn care services at various levels of public health facilities
9. Rashtriya Bal Swasthya Karyakram (RBSK)	i. Improving child health by early identification and early intervention in 4 'D's, viz., defects at birth, deficiencies, diseases, development delays including disability
10. India Newborn Action Plan (INAP)	j. Ending preventable newborn deaths to achieve "Single Digit NMR" by 2030, with all the states to individually achieve this target by 2035

Ans. 1—c, 2—a, 3—b, 4—d, 5—g, 6—e, 7—f, 8—h, 9—i, 10—j

Q3. Match the developmental test with its areas of coverage.

Test	*Domain*
1. Baroda Developmental Screening Test (BDST)	a. Mental and motor
2. Denver Developmental Screening test II (DDST)	b. Motor, language, personal, social
3. Trivandrum Developmental Screening Chart (TDSC)	c. Cognitive and motor
4. Bayley Infant Neurodevelopmental Screen (BINS)	d. Neurological processes, expressive and receptive functions, cognitive
5. Age Stage Questionnaire-3 (ASQ)	e. Motor-gross and fine, communication, problem solving, personal adaptive skills
6. Parents Evaluation of Developmental Status (PEDS)	f. Motor, vision, hearing, language and concept, self-help and social skills
7. Psychosocial developmental screening test—ICMR-PDST	g. Cognitive, motor, language, social emotional behavior, self-help, and school
8. INCLEN Neurodevelopmental Screening Tool (NDST)	h. Autism spectrum disorder (ASD), learning disorders, speech and language vision, hearing, attention-deficit/hyperactivity disorder (ADHD), delay, cerebral palsy, neuromuscular disorders, and epilepsy

Ans. 1—c, 2—b, 3—a, 4—d, 5—e, 6—g, 7—f, 8—h

Q4. Match the column.

Mechanism	*Anomaly*
1. Dysplasia	a. Down syndrome
2. Disruption	b. Amniotic band sequence
3. Deformation	c. Club foot
4. Malformation	d. Skeletal dysplasia
	e. TORCH infection

Ans. 1—d, 2—b, 3—c, 4—a

Q5. Spot the spot.

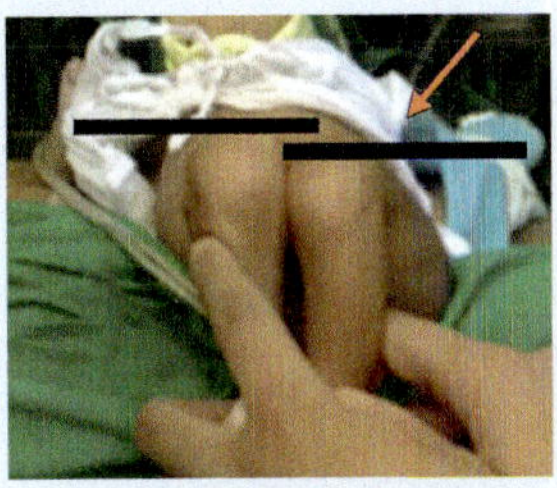

1.

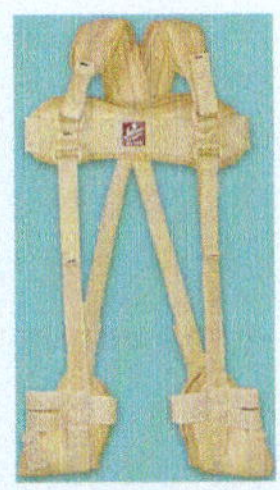

2.

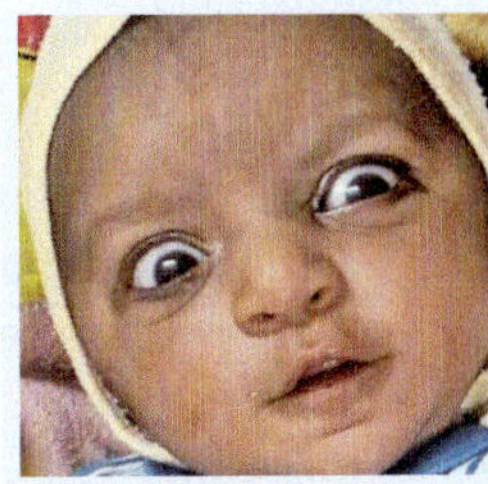

3.

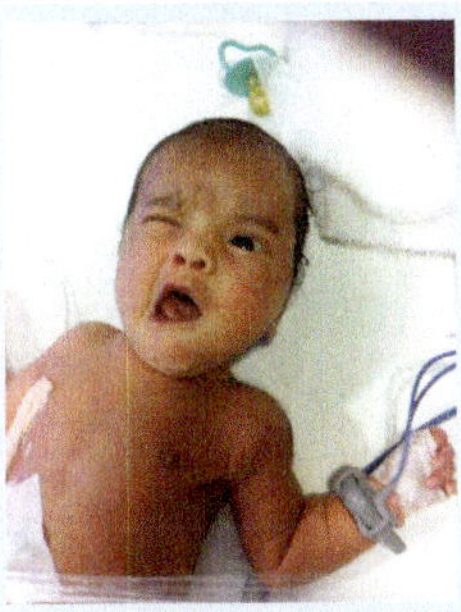

4.

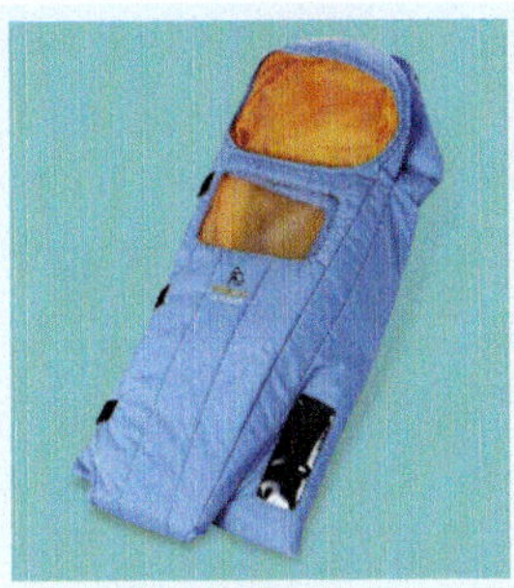

5.

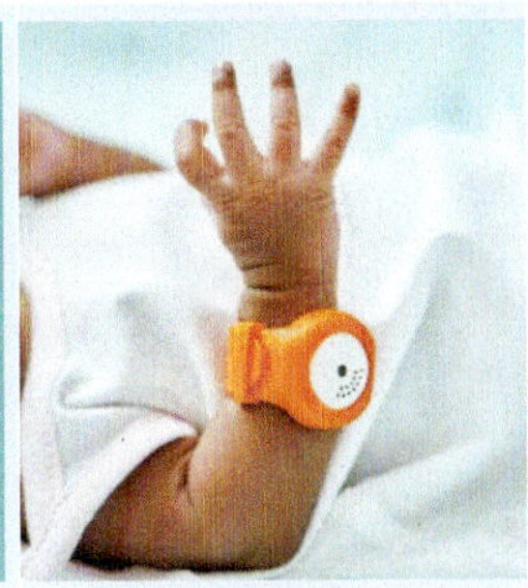

6.

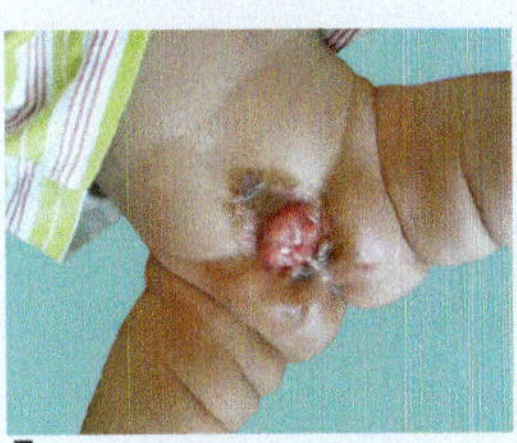

7.

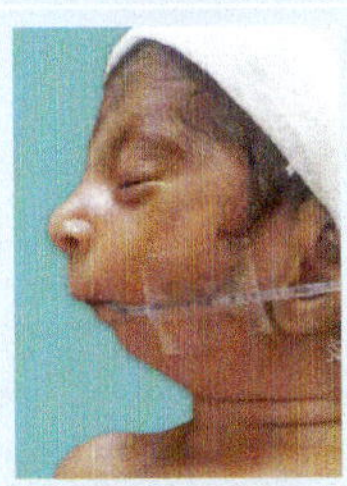

8.

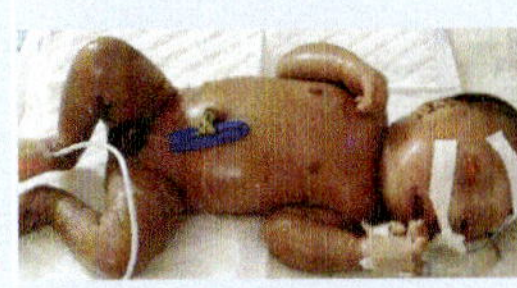

9.

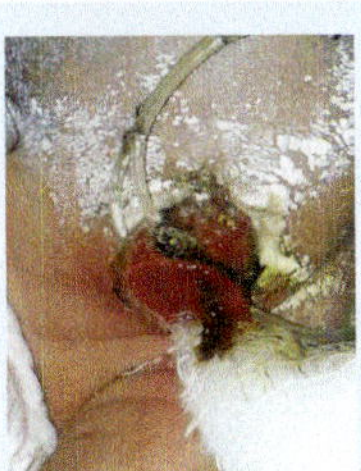

10.

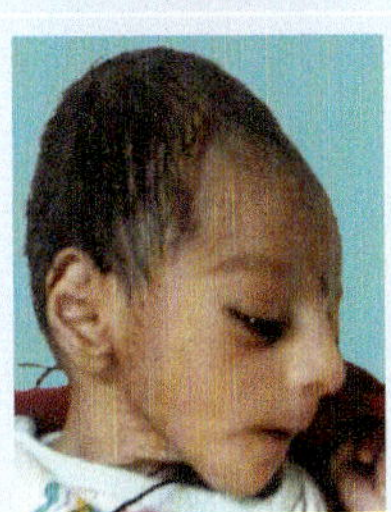

11.

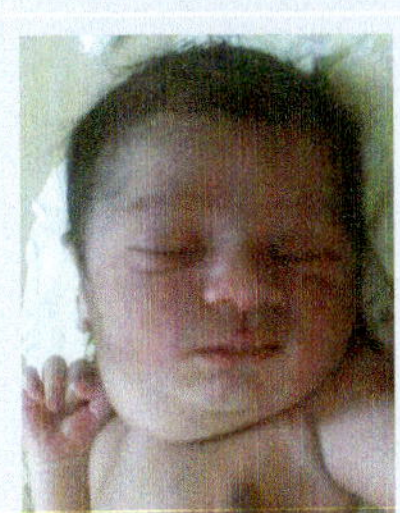

12.

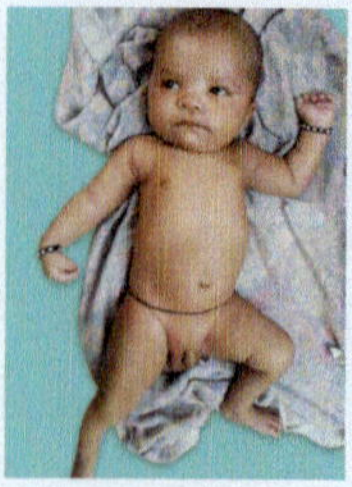

13.

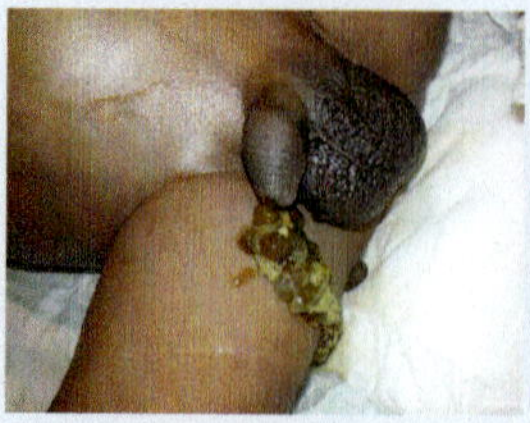

14.

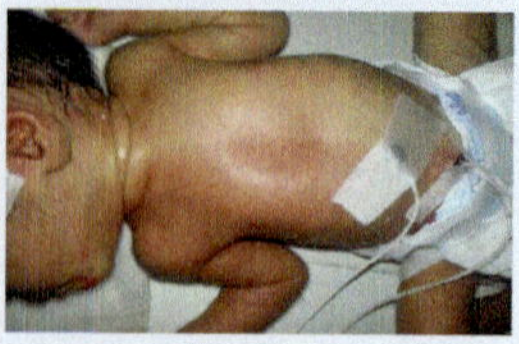

15.

Ans.

1. Galeazzi sign
2. Pavlik harness
3. Sun Set Sign
4. Absent depressor anguli oris muscle
5. Phase change portable warmer—Embrace
6. Digital temperature watch—BEMPU
7. Bladder exstrophy
8. Retrognathia
9. Collodion baby
10. Colostomy
11. Turricephaly
12. Cystic hygroma
13. Right brachial plexus injury—Klumpke's palsy
14. Recto urethral fistula
15. Harlequin skin change

Index

Page numbers followed by *f* refer to figure and *t* refer to table.

O

P

R

S

T

U

V

W

X

Z